Quantifying Quality in Primary Care

Peter Graves

Foreword by

Kieran Sweeney

Assistant Director of Policy
Commission for Health Improvement
Lecturer in General Practice and Health Services Research
Peninsula Medical School

Radcliffe Medical Press

Radcliffe Medical Press Ltd
18 Marcham Road
Abingdon
Oxon OX14 1AA
United Kingdom

www.radcliffe-oxford.com
The Radcliffe Medical Press electronic catalogue and online ordering facility.
Direct sales to anywhere in the world.

© 2002 Peter Graves

All rights reserved. No part of this publication may be reproduced, stored in a retrieval system or transmitted, in any form or by any means, electronic, mechanical, photocopying, recording or otherwise without the prior permission of the copyright owner.

British Library Cataloguing in Publication Data

A catalogue record for this book is available from the British Library.

ISBN 1 85775 599 5

Typeset by Advance Typesetting Ltd, Long Hanborough, Oxon
Printed and bound by TJ International Ltd, Padstow, Cornwall

Contents

Foreword

The last decade has seen profound changes in primary care. The profession has changed, placing evidenced practice at the centre of clinical care. Society has changed, demanding greater transparency and greater accountability. And the politicians ·have changed too, sensing this sea change in society's approach to healthcare and implementing a sweeping and radical agenda for improving the quality of care in the National Health Service.

Central to this drive for quality has been the notion of clinical governance. Initially an unfamiliar and nebulous notion – how well we remember 'the framework within which excellence can flourish' – the elements of clinical governance are now much more clearly recognised by members of the primary healthcare team. But how to do it? That's the challenge. This book, whose author has extensive experience in assessing general practice and developing practical tools for assessing quality in primary care, is a practical tool for healthcare professionals seeking to implement clinical governance. The book separates quality into three main areas – the patient's experience, patient management and practice management – and dissects each of these areas, describing in astonishing detail the range of activities appropriate for that area. Each chapter places the particular clinical activity in the context of professional, statutory or quality markers before charting, at the end of each section, an assessment map detailing specific appropriate activities. The author has been careful to avoid personal bias in selecting particular activities, helpfully referencing specific quality indicators to their programme of origin. Thus, Quality Team Development, Fellowship by Assessment of the Royal College of General Practitioners or the Quality Practice Award criteria, are clearly identified and referenced.

The level of detail in listing relevant activities under each of the three areas might appear daunting to some practices. But quality improvement does not happen overnight, and the trick will be to plan a rolling programme of improvements starting with the most pressing areas. All members of the primary healthcare team can follow the recommendations in this book. Indeed, one approach for a practice could be to delegate quality areas to groups of staff to spread the responsibilities, and to disseminate the fruits of success more widely.

The book will be helpful for all members of the primary healthcare team. It may prove particularly useful for trainers and registrars in general practice who will find it a wealth of well-referenced information about key quality activities. The author is to be commended for setting out in painstaking detail the kind of activities which practices could be recommended when seeking to improve their services for patients. For those still searching for an answer to the question, 'But just how do you do quality?', this book will be an invaluable tool.

Kieran Sweeney
Peninsula Medical School
June 2002

About the author

The author worked for 12 years in a semi-rural teaching practice in the South Midlands. As an LMC representative, he found himself on several other committees, including the 'Service Committee', and later acted as an advisor and assessor under the complaints process, which came into being in 1996, giving him experience in understanding and handling complaints.

Back at the practice, he had an interest in staff management, health and safety at work, IT systems and other aspects of clinical risk management, all of these forming some of the cornerstones of what soon became the clinical governance agenda.

In 1998, he joined an innovative, first-wave personal medical services (PMS) pilot in Central London. The pilot team consisted of a practice manager and four doctors, all qualified and trained GPs. The doctors had different degrees of experience as well as differing primary care interests: two had recently finished vocational training in Central London and had gone on to work in academic areas of primary care before joining the PMS pilot; two, including the author, had at least ten years' experience in GMS general practice. The other more experienced GP had been a trainer for many years.

The practice manager had extensive experience in hospital administration and was undertaking the Association of Medical Secretaries, Practice Administrators and Receptionists (AMSPAR) course in primary care practice management.

This team of five was employed by an acute hospital trust in Central London. The main difference between this and other PMS pilots was that it did not have a registered list of patients or any attached staff.

The aim of this pilot project was for the acute hospital trust to offer support to the local GPs in developing their services. This was done by offering free clinical and administrative input from the team. All practices were sited in a deprived part of Central London.

The local GPs submitted an application for assistance to the hospital, which outlined how they wished their practices to develop in the coming 12 months, and in what way they felt the GPs employed by the hospital might help in these developments. Practices were selected by an independent panel based on the perceived need of the practice and also the development plan submitted. Each doctor in the team was then allocated to a practice for 12 months. From the practices' point of view there were no strings attached, apart from helping evaluate the pilot scheme.

From the point of view of the team, however, it had to show to line managers that the doctors were encouraging and supporting practice development. They wanted proof that improvements in primary care services were being made.

Therefore, a question that had to be asked early in the project was how could the team show that *quality* improvements were taking place? The first part of the answer to this question was that in order to measure changes that had taken place within the year, an assessment of the starting point had to be made.

At the same time as the project started, the quality agenda within the NHS was taking off. The words 'clinical governance' were new and barely understandable, especially within the context of primary care.

During the first year of the pilot the doctors carried out a simple 'SWOT' analysis of the practices, assessing strengths, weaknesses, opportunities and threats. They wrote a plan for the practices based on the initial application plans and incorporating the SWOT analysis. For example, if a practice wanted to develop a specific disease clinic, the doctor from the team would carry out appropriate audits in the practice to assess the potential workload. Then an evidence-based protocol would be written ensuring that all those concerned with the development of the clinic were involved.

Alternatively, the team member might carry out surgeries for the existing doctors, while they did the ground work. One of the most obvious successes was with a practice that was keen to move from its existing premises into refurbished accommodation. The doctors from the team not only carried out surgeries while the partners discussed their new premises with contractors or architects, but also helped with the project management and negotiations throughout the whole process.

At the end of the first year a full report was written and presented to the line managers. At the start of the second year, however, they requested much more detail. Quantifying the quality improvements was now expected! It was at this point that the author started researching the available literature on existing assessment methods and working on a simple tool to assess the quality of services provided by practices.

During this second year, the author worked with one of the hospital departments in developing and implementing their clinical governance policies and audit programmes. The pilot finished before the tool was developed. However, the experience of evaluating the quality of management systems and their impact on patient care within practices stood the author in good stead for continuing the work as an independent consultant in several other parts of London. It was, by now, even more essential that a robust assessment tool was fully developed and evaluated. This book is the end result.

At the end of the PMS pilot, the author started working as a consultant in primary care for a London health authority. This work has involved leading on the clinical governance agenda, translating government policies into something more meaningful for GPs, and assessing and working with practices seen as 'underperforming' for whatever reason.

Towards the end of 2001, the author worked as an advisor to the Commission for Health Improvement (CHI) during the development of its primary care trust (PCT) and general practice clinical governance review tool and he became a trained clinical governance reviewer.

This book is dedicated to Ben, for whom quantity is important; to Clare, for whom quality is paramount; and to Sue, for whom 'European Excellence' is vital – but can one compare general practice with chocolate?

INTRODUCTION

Tender-handed stroke the nettle,
And it stings you for your pains:
Grasp it like a man of mettle,
And it soft as silk remains.

Aaron Hill 1685–1750

1

Quality in primary care

There are probably as many definitions of quality in healthcare systems as there are users, providers and managers of the National Health Service (NHS). Birch *et al.*[1] place these perspectives into the following categories:

- professional/medical
- lay
- managerial
- political.

To complicate the issue further, what is deemed good quality seems transitory. For example, one day a regular user of the NHS can be perfectly satisfied; the next day making a complaint. No doubt many of those who work in the NHS reading this book will identify with that. Add to that the pressures brought about by newspaper reports and television documentaries, and the issues become even less clear.

Historically, governments have measured quality in terms of waiting times, cervical smear rates and drug expenditure, and by other criteria that are easily counted or costed. Professionals, on the other hand, often express the feeling that most of these are a poor reflection of quality; and this is especially the case in general practice.

To make things more difficult for the profession, in the past ten years, successive governments have moved the goal posts. More recently we have seen a shift from persistent cost cutting and 'number crunching' to an improvement of quality and health outcomes, although political views of quality often appear very different to medical or professional views.

In the past five years, the current government has focused very closely on quality. The term 'clinical governance' was coined in the government's White Paper, *The New NHS: modern, dependable*.[2] It is this clinical governance agenda that has been the driver for many changes in the NHS, including the delivery of primary care. The White Paper was followed by a series of National Service Frameworks (NSFs) and many health service guidance papers on quality initiatives, which focus on outcomes by enhancing the quality of healthcare delivery. Primary care has diligently taken most of these initiatives on board. Furthermore, as medical knowledge grows and technology advances, the NHS has even greater pressure to deliver optimal, up-to-date medical care.

A classical example of political and research pressures combined is the flu vaccination programmes. Up until the early 1990s, there was little evidence that flu vaccine really provided an adequate, cost-effective mechanism for protecting populations from influenza. Now target payments are being paid to GPs to vaccinate the over-65s.

Initiatives like these put further pressure on general practice to provide an effective, efficient service. Recent changes in the way primary care is delivered have been attempts to improve access as well as delivery, and the new locally negotiated personal medical services (PMS) contracts and 'walk-in centres' are good examples of this.

Chapter 10 of the White Paper, *The New NHS: modern, dependable* promises patients that their views will be 'represented within the NHS'. We are, therefore, committed to include the 'customers'' views when planning healthcare systems. The real question that needs asking is, 'Have we been able to improve health outcomes in general practice?'

There are many excellent books written by academics and health workers about their definitions of quality and clinical governance in health services. Many of these are researched, evidence-based and very theoretical; few have practical suggestions for busy practices of methods of improving quality and putting clinical governance principles into primary care. This book fills that gap by giving the reader guidance on how to assess general practice. It offers suggestions of how quality improvements may be achieved.

Assessment: the first step

If clinical governance reviewers from the Commission for Health Improvement (CHI) turned up on the doorstep of the practice today, what would they find? Indeed, how would they assess the practice and what would they be looking for? This book aims to answer those questions and direct anyone who has to assess quality in everyday general practice towards answering the question, 'What are good quality services in primary care?' It should be as easy for GPs, practice managers and practice nurses to use as managers of health authorities and primary care trusts (PCTs).

The experiences of patients accessing primary care services can be significantly influenced by the efficiency of the systems within the practice. The practice manager and staff are essential to the smooth running of primary care in the 21st century, and the appropriate training and overall attitude of the staff is, ultimately, the responsibility of the doctors. The clinical care that takes place in general practice day in, day out is underpinned by complex administrative processes. However good the clinical care may be, if the administrative processes fail, patients can still be put at risk.

Those doctors and managers who have to deal with practices considered to be 'underperforming' freely admit that it is rare to find a doctor whose clinical knowledge is poor while the systems run perfectly. It is much more the case that 'underperformance' of the systems leads to poor quality and complaints, rather than the lack of clinical knowledge of the practitioners, although this too can be wanting in some cases.

Is all this really necessary?

When you last flew off to some far country, either on a holiday or for a business trip, did you stop and think about the necessary managerial structures and administrative processes it had taken to get the aircraft safely into the sky and to the right destination in one piece? Did you consider whether the mechanic who last serviced the essential fuel valve followed the written procedure? Did you consider in which language the pilot might speak to the air-traffic controller on arrival? Probably not! You assumed that the appropriate protocols and procedures were followed; that the pilot and air-traffic controller spoke the same language. Yet, if the flight was delayed or altered at the last minute for 'technical reasons', you probably became somewhat annoyed, especially if the explanation was unsatisfactory.

When you start to ask questions about how much we all rely on the integrity of 'systems' and management protocols, then you should also start to question those systems that the practice is responsible for; those that others rely on, particularly patients.

As GPs, how often do we run late or cancel a surgery for 'technical reasons' with insufficient explanation to patients and then wonder why they get angry and annoyed or make a complaint? Ask yourself:

• How easy is it to get a repeat prescription?
• When were the staff last appraised?

This book guides you through these and many other questions to help you make a valued judgement of the quality of primary care management systems in the practice you are assessing. It aims to highlight many of the legal obligations held by GPs. It points out many of the obligations found in the Regulations, 1992, and subsequent amendments. I recognise that the General Medical Services (GMS) Regulations 1992 are slowly but surely being relegated and taken over by an anxiously awaited, newly negotiated contract with the government and locally negotiated PMS contracts; but it is likely that many of the principles in the GMS regulations will exist in these contracts. The guidance for development of PMS contracts has also been incorporated into many parts.

The book also predicts some aspects of the revalidation process which is rapidly approaching, which, we are told, will be based on the General Medical Council's (GMC) document *Good Medical Practice*. It outlines criteria recognised as good practice and high-quality systems. Most essentially, this book helps the reader to focus on the signs of good quality, safe patient care.

Is it relevant?

In March 1999, the government published its White Paper *Modernising Government*.[3] This set out a long-term programme of improvement in public services. It states that, 'we will deliver efficient, high-quality public services and **will not tolerate mediocrity**'.

Part of this agenda for modernisation of public services has been based on two management assessment models, 'best practice' and the 'European Excellence Model'. Local authorities, police and probation services around the country are already using these to openly evaluate service provision followed by a programme of modernisation and upgrading of services. The two models both depend on self-assessment of services provided and both have a strong 'customer' focus, as well as a results focus.

It is likely, therefore, that the NHS will follow suit, sooner or later. In fact, some acute trusts have already adopted the European Excellence Model and started a programme of self-assessment with 'customer' input. They have seen tangible improvements in service delivery.

I would argue, therefore, that to be able to carry out an in-depth evaluation of one's own practice will become an imperative.

Basis of the tool

Work in practice is now tightly regulated. On top of the NHS (GMS) regulations, there is a minefield of legislation that affects general practice, for example the laws surrounding the Health and Safety at Work Act (1974), Control of Substances Hazardous to Health (CoSHH) Regulations, Employment Laws and others.

While some GPs have opted for locally negotiated PMS contracts, it remains the case that most GPs are still bound under the National Health Service (General Medical Services) Regulations 1992 and the terms of service contained within these regulations to provide certain services. (At the time of writing this book we anxiously await a 'new contract'.) General practices are small businesses and employers, and as such are bound by partnership and employment laws.

It is these legal obligations, the management systems and the 'smooth running' of practices, among other aspects of the care you offer, that the CHI clinical governance reviewer will assess.

This book is designed as a simple, user-friendly guide to help *anyone* who has need to assess and evaluate the way practices interpret their legal obligations; the way the management systems within practices run; and the quality of the systems and processes that most affect the patient care. It is hoped that GPs will use the book as a tool to assess their own practice processes to identify those systems that are working well, those that could be improved and any essential ones that are missing altogether. Once aware of the quality and efficiency of the processes that underpin clinical care, it should be possible to build necessary improvements into a business plan focused on continued development. By using the scoring system, it is envisaged that one could prioritise future developments of practice policies and protocols. The book also contains many frameworks on which to build policies for the smooth running of practices.

The GMC is very clear on its views about 'good medical practice'; these are published in a series of pamphlets of that title and are also posted on the GMC website (www.gmc-uk.org). There is no doubt that revalidation of doctors will be based on the principles of good medical practice.

In November 2000, the Royal College of General Practitioners (RCGP) and the General Practitioners Committee (GPC) of the British Medical Association (BMA) published a draft document, *Good Medical Practice for General Practitioners*. This put the GMC's documents into a primary care perspective. It clearly laid out acceptable and unacceptable practices.

Furthermore, mechanisms for assessment and accreditation by the RCGP for quality services provided by practices have been in existence for some time. These include quality team development (QTD) and quality practice award (QPA), both designed as quality assessments and development programmes of the whole primary healthcare team (PHCT).

Individual GPs have also been able to gain recognition of high-quality practice by achieving Membership or Fellowship of the RCGP by Assessment of Performance (MAP and FBA respectively). The criteria for achieving these are now well established and continue to be evaluated and adjusted annually. Details of the criteria, along with application forms, can be obtained from the RCGP.

Shortly after starting the process of developing this tool, the Scottish Board published its criteria for revalidation of practices.

This tool to assess practices has been written and evaluated with all these in mind. It covers many areas of primary care, and the answers to the questions posed provide a clear insight into the attitudes of those working within practices. It has now been used in many practices, ranging from excellent practices offering a wide range of high-quality services to those that have significant areas for improvement. All practices feel that they have benefited from a structured assessment and the objective result. All have been able to show areas where further practice development can be made. Evaluation of good systems has, in itself, allowed practices to learn what makes the system run well and ask, 'How can this be utilised to develop other systems?'

Some practices have been able to formulate prioritised plans for the future in order to consider a PMS bid or to put a good business case to the primary care organisation for further developmental assistance. The value of self-assessment in such depth is enormous.

While the areas covered are extensive, I have no doubt that there will be those who feel that the most essential feature of quality in their practice is missing, and there will be those that feel it is too detailed. The areas included are those the author has found most useful for practices themselves and for informing PCTs. Frequently, when assessing a practice, one or more of the included areas opens up discussion about a related topic not included in the tool; the starting point, however, was one area assessed by this tool. Don't be blinkered by the questions asked, or the areas focused on, allow other areas to be included in the assessment using the same principles found here.

One health authority used part of the tool to assist in the decision-making process for how best to help a practitioner who faced losing his practice when the senior partner retired. An inner-London PCT has used the repeat prescribing section to develop a repeat prescribing audit tool as part of its prescribing incentive scheme.

I would strongly advise that the parts of the tool are used one at a time, focusing on single aspects of a practice in order to make adjustments and improvements and then returning at a later date to reassess that change before moving on to another area. Furthermore, the involvement of the entire PHCT in answering some of the questions and discussing the results should make the experience of evaluation more valuable and probably more objective. It is likely that involvement of the whole team will enhance team relationships, encourage new ideas and bring out better solutions for problem solving.

Experience shows that the more involved team members are in the development of the practice, the more loyal and interested they are in achieving favourable outcomes. It can certainly be an excellent way to prove what hard work goes on in practices and praise those members whose input is vital but not always recognised as such.

If it stimulates debate, guides those working with or in primary care towards ideas to enhance the way services are delivered and, ultimately, improves outcomes for patients, then it has achieved the author's aims for writing the book.

References

1   Birch K, Field S, Scrivens E (2000) *Quality in General Practice*. Radcliffe Medical Press, Oxford.

2   Department of Health (1998) *The New NHS: modern, dependable*. The Stationery Office, London.

3   Cabinet Office (1999) *Modernising Government*. The Stationery Office, London.

2

Using the tool

> **Aims of the tool**
>
> To assist in making an objective assessment of general practices in order to help practices develop sound processes and administrative systems, thereby enhancing the quality of patient care in line with clinical governance and evidence-based principles. The assessment should allow practices to:
>
> - develop and promote those processes and systems that are working well
> - evaluate those that are not working so well and decide which should be improved and which should be replaced
> - discover those gaps in service delivery which should be addressed urgently.

At the end of each chapter there is a table of questions to be answered by the assessor. The first column on the left indicates whether the criterion being assessed is:

- a legal requirement (L)
- a 'Terms of Service'[1] or PMS contractual requirement (ToS)
- considered an essential requirement by the GMC[2] and emphasised in *Good Medical Practice for General Practitioners*[3] (E) (criteria under this category are likely to form part of the assessment for revalidation)
- considered good practice in *Good Medical Practice for GPs* (G)
- an RCGP Quality Team Development criterion (QTD)
- essential for Membership by Assessment of Performance of the Royal College of GPs (MAP) – April 2001
- essential for Fellowship by Assessment of the Royal College of GPs (FBA) – April 2001, 12th version.

The boxes in the second column contain a question about a system being assessed. The last three columns contain answers to the questions posed or suggested standards by which a system can be measured, rather like a multiple choice exam paper. Each answer should be a guide to help evaluate the system in place. The boxes in the final three columns can be completed in one of two ways.

The first is simply to tick the boxes which most accurately answers the question.

- A tick in the first box indicates that the system works badly or doesn't exist.
- A tick in the second box indicates that the system works but needs reviewing and updating or the standard could be better.
- A tick in the third box indicates that the system is working as well as it should or a high standard is met.

It is strongly suggested that you add a comment under each answer to explain why you answered the way you did, for your future reference. This will be especially useful if the process of assessment is carried out again in the future.

Remember, the validity of the tool is dependent on consistency and honesty. If you continually try to put yourself in the position of a patient by asking the question, 'If I were a patient using services at this practice how would I wish to be treated?', you may find that your answers reflect the true situation *and not the one you think is in place*. Furthermore, the more members of staff you involve in answering the questions, the more likely you are to get the truth. As a bonus, the involvement of the entire PHCT is likely to enhance teamwork.

After completing each section, the assessor can then count the ticks in each column. On returning to re-evaluate each system, you compare the scores. The aim, of course, is to increase the overall number of ticks in the last column.

Alternatively, it is possible to refine the scoring system and differentiate within each box, evaluating not only how well it works but also reflecting the importance of the system. In each of the boxes containing the answers, there are three further boxes containing a score. Higher scores reveal that important and essential systems are working well. The lower the score, the more urgently it must be reviewed.

Scores range from 1 to 3 in the first box, 4 to 6 in the second box and 7 to 9 in the third. The assessor then judges a question being asked on its degree of importance or urgency and grades the score given accordingly.

An example might be to evaluate the Health and Safety at Work policy. The scoring system might look like this:

Health and Safety at Work policy

L	Does the practice have a **Health and Safety policy**? (a legal requirement if there are five or more employees)	No, but we should have one No, because there are fewer than five employees	Yes, but it is the one sent by the health authority and has not been adapted to suit the practice situation	Yes, it has been locally developed. The practice is well aware of the importance of a Health and Safety policy and does not just have one because it is a legal requirement Despite having fewer than five employees there is still a Health and Safety policy because the practice is aware of the relevance and importance of having such a policy
		Score 1 / Score 2 / Score 3	Score 4 / Score 5 / Score 6	Score 7 / Score 8 / Score 9

In the first box:

- A score of 1 could denote that the practice has no Health and Safety at Work policy at all. Because it is a legal requirement (for practices employing more than five staff) it should be developed urgently. Therefore a tick should be placed in score box 1. If there are fewer than five employees, there is no legal obligation to have a Health and Safety at Work policy, but it would be good practice to have one. As such, the urgency placed on this is less (from a legal viewpoint) but still important. A score of 3 would be reasonable.

In the second column:

- A score of 4 could denote that the Health and Safety at Work policy is really only the guidance pack that was sent by the health authority and has not been locally adapted. What's more, the staff are unaware that it exists. This should be addressed *soon* but not immediately. If the staff were aware of aspects of the policy it would be reasonable to score slightly higher, say 5.

In the third column:

- A score of 7 means that the Health and Safety at Work policy is locally adapted to suit the practice's situation and while the staff are aware of its existence, they are not regularly appraised in its importance and usage. Perhaps you have not had a fire drill for several years. In other words, the system runs well but needs a little improvement.

Another example might be the staff appraisal system.

Staff appraisals

G	Do staff regularly undergo appraisals?	No			Yes, but the process is not linked with the practice development plan			Yes, staff are encouraged to discuss their own needs during the appraisal and these are linked in with the practice development plan and needs of the practice, in order that the practice can continue to offer more comprehensive services		
		Score 1	Score 2	Score 3	Score 4	Score 5	Score 6	Score 7	Score 8	Score 9

- A score of 3 in the first box could denote that the staff have never had individual appraisals. While a staff appraisal system is good practice, it isn't a legal requirement and can take a lower precedence over other legal requirements.
- A score of 5 in the second box denotes that staff are appraised but appraisals don't really address the needs of the staff or the practice. As it stands it is not a priority to alter it, but both staff and practice could benefit from improvements.
- A score of 8 means that the system is nearly perfect; for example, the staff views are taken into account and their requests for training listened to, but these don't always fit into the practice development plan.

One further example might be the complaints system. This is a requirement under NHS regulations and, therefore, should work efficiently.

- The fact that a practice doesn't have a complaints procedure and an indication that there is antagonism towards patients that make comments or complaints would warrant a maximum score of 2.
- Should the practice use the complaints procedure sent to them by a health authority in 1996 when the new complaints procedure came into being, and this works in terms of replying to the patients within the appropriate time limits, but there isn't a true understanding of how to resolve complaints and learn from them, then this would score 6 at the most.

- A score of 9 in the third box means that an audit of the system showed that the system runs as perfectly as can be expected; a review in one year will show it continues to function just as well. For example, the complaints system adheres to the NHS guidelines that the few complaints received have been resolved to the full satisfaction of the patients as well as the doctors. A patient may even have complimented you about how well a complaint was handled.

By having a more detailed and differential scoring system you are likely to gain from the assessment. Furthermore, you will be able to assess progress more satisfactorily at a later date. If a more complex system of scoring is adopted, it is essential that you write notes and comments to remind yourself why you scored the question the way you did. If it scored well, you should comment on why the system was running well; for example, were there specific personnel who made it run well? What lessons can be learned to utilise in other systems?

If you scored a system somewhat lower, comment on why you thought the system did not reach the standard you felt it should, and in what way you envisage improvements could be made. It might take longer to carry out, but the more thorough the assessment, the more valuable it will be in the long run. If other staff are involved they will need to be well briefed before starting to ensure consistency.

At the end of each chart you should total up the number of areas scoring 1, 2 or 3 – these urgently need to be put in place or significantly improved. Then the number of areas scoring 4, 5 or 6, which need reviewing and improving. And finally, the number of areas scoring 7, 8 or 9. These are working well – ask yourself, 'Can the principles of these systems be transferred to other areas of practice work?' Repeat the questions in a few months' time to assess and quantify how much improvement the practice has achieved in the quality of the service and systems.

The areas covered in the book are divided into three main areas:

1   The patients' experience
    - Chapter 4 Access
    - Chapter 5 Building, environment and equipment
2   Patient management and treatment
    - Chapter 6 Health promotion and chronic disease management
    - Chapter 7 Prescribing
    - Chapter 8 Record keeping and letters
3   Practice management policies, staff and education
    - Chapter 9 Management policies, clinical governance and risk management
    - Chapter 10 Staff employment
    - Chapter 11 Communication and team working
    - Chapter 12 IT and computerised systems
    - Chapter 13 Continuing medical education and personal professional development

References

1   *The National Health Service (General Medical Services) Regulations 1992.* HMSO, London.

2   General Medical Council (1998) *Good Medical Practice* (2e). GMC, London.

3   General Practitioners Committee and Royal College of General Practitioners (2000) *Good Medical Practice for General Practitioners*. GPC and RCGP, London.

PART ONE
THE PATIENTS' EXPERIENCE

Honest labour bears a lovely face.

Thomas Dekker 1572–1632

3

Practice demography

It is surprising that assessments of practices often reveal that they have little idea of their true demography. It would seem ludicrous for a private company to be offering a service without having a very good idea of its customer base. Few ice-cream van owners, for example, are found in areas where there are no children during the winter!

In this day and age when at the press of a button one can print out an age–sex distribution of the practice patient list, there is little excuse for not doing so.

> The age–sex distribution of one practice assessed showed that they had 12% of their practice under the age of 10 and 22% under the age of 20. Of the 12% under the age of 10, 60% were under 5. The practice had difficulty in achieving vaccination targets and, what is more, the one-hour baby clinic on Thursday afternoon was described as 'a nightmare'. The relationship with the health visitors was frosty to say the least.
>
> As the doctors were unaware of the high proportion of children they had registered with them, they hadn't considered redistributing time accordingly.
>
> Suggestions to address this included employing a PMS doctor to focus on providing child health services and aiming to become a paediatric GP specialist.

Some time to assess the demography of the practice, and genuinely ask whether the service provided focuses on those that need healthcare the most, is valuable. A high elderly population, for example, may need a coordinated regular visiting timetable, with the visits distributed by geography between the doctors, district nurses and health visitors. If this can be integrated with the over-75 annual check (paragraph 16 of Terms of Service) and the flu vaccine programme, the system will be efficient and cost-effective. There is no reason why this obvious work pressure cannot be included in a PMS contract bid.

It seems a waste of resources (mainly manpower) to be providing an excellent contraceptive clinic in the middle of the afternoon if there are very few women in their late teens, twenties and thirties who can actually get to it.

Similarly, assess the deprivation payments. If these are relatively high, this can be used as a lever to persuade the PCT or local health group (LHG in Wales) to provide other services at the surgery; for example, a visiting benefits advisor or social worker.

Bearing in mind that diabetes, coronary heart disease and other chronic illnesses affect ethnic groups differently,[1] consider how well the practice knows the ethnic distribution of the population. Should the screening programmes be more targeted to those in the higher-risk groups? The government intends to set targets for practices to know their ethnic distribution. If the practice isn't already doing so, it should consider collecting the data for all new patients now.

Furthermore, it is well recognised that some service users specifically prefer to see professionals of one gender. For example, some women, for personal or religious reasons, will only consult female doctors or nurses. In areas of high ethnic numbers, adequate provision must be made for this or practices will not hit cervical screening targets and the health of the population will suffer as a result.

Health authority public health departments should be able to provide practices with demographic and ethnic data. The department will also have statistical evidence about disease prevalence in the area. The practice can then make logical, evidence-based decisions about service provision for the future.

Other demographic considerations might include:

- local industries – are there work-related illnesses associated with local industry?
- level of unemployment
- accessibility to services – particularly relevant in rural settings.

Key question

• Are there examples of where the practice has made significant changes to the service provision on the grounds of demographic information?

References

1 The Runnymede Trust (2000) *The Future of Multi-Ethnic Britain*. The Parek Report 2000, chaired by Bhikhu Parekh.
2 Census 2001; race and ethnic categories.

List size

Age–sex distribution										
Age	0–9	10–19	20–29	30–39	40–49	50–59	60–69	70–79	80–89	90+
Females										
% total										
Males										
% total										
Totals										
% total										

Demography

- Rural
- Inner city
- Sub-urban
- Mixed.

Practice profile

	Number	Comments, e.g. whole time equivalents, interests in primary care and outside interests
Principals		
Assistants		

Other doctors		
Practice nurses		
Practice manager		
Deputy		
Receptionists		
Secretary		
Computer data inputter		
Other staff		
Attached staff and allied health professionals		
District nurses		
Health visitors		
Midwife		
Physiotherapist		
Chiropractor		
Chiropodist		
Counsellor		
Others		

Deprivation payments	Level 1	Level 2	Level 3	Level 4

Ethnicity[2] (2001 census categories)	Females	Males	Total
White: British			
White: Irish			
White: Other			
Mixed: White and Black Caribbean			
Mixed: White and Black African			
Mixed: White and Asian			
Asian or Asian British: Indian			
Asian or Asian British: Pakistani			
Asian or Asian British: Bangladeshi			
Asian or Asian British: Other			
Black or Black British: Caribbean			
Black or Black British: African			
Black or Black British: Other			
Chinese			
Other ethnic group			
Refusal			

4

Access

Background

Access to healthcare has been recognised as one of the measures of quality of healthcare systems since the 1980s. In 1984, Robert Maxwell[1] took Avedis Donabedian's three inter-related components of quality assessment[2] of health services – goodness, effectiveness and environment (sometimes referred to as the triad: Processes, Outcomes and Structure) – and identified six core components of his own, namely:

- effectiveness
- acceptability
- efficiency
- equity
- relevance
- access.

In terms of access, he asked the obvious question, 'Can people get treatment when and where they need it?' Successive governments have focused on improved access to primary care services as a way to improve healthcare.

In 1992, the Conservative Government made changes in the regulations governing GMS GPs, which were prescriptive in terms of the numbers of hours GPs spent consulting patients. Since then a full-time GMS GP has had to spend no fewer than 26 hours each week 'normally available to provide such services'. What is more, these have to be spread over five days of the week. A three-quarter time doctor can spend fewer than 26 hours but not fewer than 19 hours each week and a half-time doctor fewer than 19 hours but not fewer than 13 hours each week 'available' (Regulation 15 of the NHS (GMS) Regulations 1992).

Further, GMS GPs must be available to their patients no fewer than 42 weeks per year (paragraph 29, (2) (a), NHS (GMS) Regulations 1992).

Doctors who have negotiated a PMS contract may have negotiated different systems for access. Access to services may be more 'integrated', and take into account other professionals and local providers like walk-in centres, and it is likely that access to the GPs is based on the same principles and they will need to be available to consult for very similar periods of time in order to achieve agreed targets.

It is difficult to believe that access is still very difficult for some service users in the UK.

During one assessment of a practice in London, the appointments book was reviewed. Two months during 2000 were randomly chosen to assess availability.

On average, the doctor started consulting at 11.00am and finished about noon. The GP then started again at 4.00pm and finished at 5.00pm. On Thursday afternoon the GP took a half-day! During the two months assessed, the average face-to-face consulting was 9½ hours per week.

The doctor was witnessed spending over two hours per day writing acute prescriptions for patients who had left messages with the receptionist. Interestingly, the GP complained that patients were becoming more and more demanding!

Since the introduction of these regulations in 1992, there has been some considerable controversy about what 'normally available to provide such services' really means. The government fought for it to mean face-to-face contact time. The profession insisted that so much time was spent on paperwork and other patient-related activities that these should also be taken into account.

Initially, practices were expected to provide the health authority with timetables of the actual time spent in surgery, in order that they could check that doctors were spending the appropriate amount of time consulting with patients in line with their contractual obligations. Timetables of doctors' consulting times are still a requirement in the practice leaflet under the GMS Terms of Service regulations.

In reality, many health authorities allowed a period of time each day for visiting and some patient-related paperwork, reducing the surgery times down to about 21 hours for full-time doctors. Furthermore, doctors were allowed to do other 'health-related' activity for at least one session per week, allowing a little more flexibility.

Improving access to primary care services has been high on this government's agenda ever since its election in 1996. In the publication on the UK National Service Framework, *A First Class Service: quality in the New NHS* (1998),[3] the second on the list of the six quality criteria was 'fair access'.

Since then the NHS Plan, published in July 2000, gave a target that by 2004, patients should be able to access a primary care professional within 24 hours and a GP within 48 hours. Chapter 12 reads:

> In future all practices will be required to guarantee this level of access for their patients, either by providing it themselves, or by entering into an arrangement with another practice ...[4]

It hasn't just been the government, however, that considers fair access to services as a marker of quality; the GMC in paragraph 31 of *Good Medical Practice* says that the team must understand the need to provide 'responsive and accessible and effective service'.

Likewise, the RCGP assesses availability as part of its quality assessments and accreditation. Practices have to submit evidence of availability to the assessors, which is later confirmed.

There are many aspects to access that need consideration by GPs.

Access to professionals

Patients expect to be able to get appointments to see their GP at their convenience, whenever necessary, 24 hours a day, 365 days of the year. A constant criticism by service users is the difficulty they have in getting appointments, or the fact that the telephone lines are frequently engaged.

Some high street supermarkets are now open 24 hours a day or seven days a week. In contrast, many GP surgeries not only close for a half a day during the week, but many still close for several hours at lunchtime and don't open at all at weekends. For commuters therefore, it is nearly impossible to gain access to services without taking time off work. This is a situation that many resent and arguably leads to inadequate healthcare for significantly large groups of people.

Should GPs consider addressing these problems of access, or are these problems that governments should provide answers for? Clearly, initiatives like walk-in centres and NHS Direct are the first signs that the government is providing back-up services to general practice to assist in solving the problem of access to primary care services, but these too have their critics. The walk-in centres in central London have proved very popular and early statistics reveal that as many as 40% of those using walk-in centres aren't registered with a GP (personal correspondence).

This, however, isn't the only aspect of access to be considered.

Out-of-hours access

Access to care outside normal surgery hours is an essential part of the service that practices have to provide, either themselves or by making alternative arrangements for emergency cover. The detail of how emergency care is obtained by patients differs from practice to practice. More and more frequently, however, practices are using GP cooperatives or deputising services.

The government aims that by 2004, a single telephone call to NHS Direct will access all out-of-hours providers for primary care and social services. Directing patients to the out-of-hours providers has certainly moved on from the time when the doctor's wife was expected to track the doctor down during nights and week-ends. We usually rely on the latest technological advances: answer machines, mobile phones, sophisticated pagers, automatic re-routing systems or direct computer links in our cars. How reliable are all these systems? There is no doubt that we are more accessible than we were even five or six years ago.

I remember an evening on call in the summer of 1988.

My pager went off. I had just left a patient and was not inclined to return to ask to use their telephone to call my wife to collect the next visit. I found a telephone box. It had been vandalised and as such was unserviceable. I drove to another; I was familiar enough with the geography of telephone boxes in those days! I got through easily enough, but the coin box was full and wouldn't take my 10p piece! I drove to the next. It was out of order.

By the sixth phone box and nearly an hour later I was so close to home, I simply went home to retrieve the message, whereupon I had to drive back to within yards of my previous visit.

A few weeks later I persuaded the practice to invest in our first 'mobile' phone. It was a very large, heavy piece of equipment that cost us £1200! An invaluable asset at that time, I still maintain.

Other services

Primary care is being expected to provide access to a wide range of diverse services. The questions in this chapter cover the accessibility to and the quality of some of these other services. They include obstetric care, child health surveillance and minor surgery services, counselling, links to social services and many more.

A more detailed assessment of immunisation programmes and for women is included in the health promotion section of Chapter 6.

Telephone access

Many surgeries allocate a period of time during the day when patients can access the doctors and nurses by telephone. Patients with difficulties accessing services can then discuss problems over the phone to request a simple service or decide whether they need to see a member of the team during surgery.

How many telephone lines are there coming into the practice? If the single or very few telephone lines coming into the practice are blocked by patients requesting routine appointments or repeat prescriptions, how do patients with emergency problems get through?

Consider a busy Monday morning. Many patients with significant problems will wait until Monday so that they don't have to 'bother the doctor' over the weekend. Do they then find they can't get through Monday morning either? British Telecom can audit the number of calls that fail to get through because the lines are busy. Some practices allow access by fax machine, for example requesting repeat prescriptions, others will respond to questions via e-mail systems.

There are many other aspects of access to primary care services that practices have to consider. Some patients need to be able to obtain specific services on a regular basis, such as obtaining certificates or repeat prescriptions. Patients have the right under the Data Protection Act to access their clinical notes. These also need consideration and careful management.

The issue of access is so important that the government has supported an initiative called 'Advanced Access in Primary Care', pioneered by the National Primary Care Development Team, Manchester.

The principle is that practices work out their day-to-day demand throughout the week then match this with capacity. It also introduces many other ways for patients to access healthcare and supports the fact that there are many professionals who can advise patients: seeing the doctor is only one.

The result is that clinical staff know that each morning they will walk into a surgery in the morning where there are enough appointments available for all those patients that request one.

The effect for practices that have participated in the programme has been very positive indeed. Not only are most patients and service users seen on the day they wish, but the stress levels for receptionists and clinical staff have dropped dramatically. I would highly recommend that any practice feeling overwhelmed with patient demand visits the website as a minimum, www.npdt.org.

Access for those with disabilities

Patients with special needs, visual, hearing and physical disabilities, those with communication impairments and those with mental health difficulties and learning disabilities, need individual consideration. Part 3 of the Disability Discrimination Act (1995) comes into force from October 2004. It covers all service provision and the physical environment needs to be adapted by October 2004. It requires that service providers ensure that the following are in place:

- easily read, colour-coded signs to highlight surgery features, even brightly coloured door frames
- better lighting
- reserved parking, and obstacle-free surgery entrances, grab rails and ramps for those with disabilities
- easy access for wheelchair users, with wide doorways
- disabled toilet facilities
- induction loops and better visual call signs
- information on tape, as well as in Braille
- better training and disability awareness for staff.

Access by those with language difficulties

In many parts of the country, particularly inner cities, doctors have many patients on their lists for whom English is not their first language. For example, in parts of London, doctors find that they have lists on which as many as 90% of the patients are Bengali-speaking, many of whom will speak no English at all. In such areas, the practice staff may reflect the local ethnic mix.

While it is tempting to use them as translators, this can lead to difficulties. Properly trained interpreters will translate as precisely as possible what the doctor or patient is saying, without prejudice or personal bias. Untrained practice staff may know the patient personally or have regular contact with them in the role of receptionist or telephonist and have biased views about the frequency of presentation or severity of the problem. This may mean that they might not translate directly and may add their own interpretation. They may also offer advice about the problem, which the doctor is unaware of. Furthermore, it may put the receptionist into a difficult position regarding patient confidentiality.

There may also be an issue about the staff member's contract and job description, which may not include acting in the capacity of translator, for which they are not adequately qualified.

Some practices have access to qualified interpreters for a specific day of the week and, therefore, run clinics on this day for patients who speak little or no English. Furthermore, most health authorities now provide telephone interpreting services available throughout the working day. They are often accessible outside normal working hours as well.

Access to information

Access to information is also important. Since 1992, practices have had to produce a practice leaflet for patients. It should contain specific details of the services provided (paragraph 47 of the Terms of Service, schedule 2 of the NHS (GMS) Regulations 1992). Schedule 12 of the NHS (GMS) Regulations specifies which 20 pieces of information should be given to patients in the practice leaflet; a timetable of availability is one of them.

The new PMS contract guidelines aren't as prescriptive as the GMS regulations, but infer that practices should provide useful information leaflets, not just an out-of-date statutory document.

Access to health records

The Data Protection Act allows patients access to their own health records. Practices must now make patients' notes available to them. They can make a small charge for this service, especially if patients want copies of their notes. This has serious implications for what is written in the records and potentially the doctor–patient relationship. All the same, it is a now a legal obligation.

The NHS Plan also promises that in the future, patients will have:

- copies of letters between clinicians about their healthcare
- smart cards, allowing access to health records.

Chapter 10 of the NHS Plan describes how patients will have far more access to information about treatments and services available and as a result will be 'empowered' by having far more choice. NHS Direct, the 'Expert Patient' programme and guidelines published by the CHI will provide some information for patients about treatments and services available.

By asking the questions relevant to accessibility, this chapter should help you to assess whether the practice is comparable to others in terms of access. Some specific services, which could be classified under the heading 'access', are covered in later chapters. The questions here relate to accessibility of doctors and other professionals in the surgery.

Try to consider the questions from the *patients' viewpoint*.

Key questions

- How easy is it to access the services from a doctor or other health professional?
- Is the practice committed to providing information about access to services?

References

1 Maxwell RJ (1984) Quality assessment in health. *BMJ*. **288**: 1470–2.

2 Donabedian A (1980) *Explorations in Quality Assessment and Monitoring, vol 1: The Definition of Quality and Approaches to its Assessment*. Health Administration Press.

3 Department of Health (1988) *A First Class Service*. The Stationery Office, London.

4 Department of Health (2000) *The NHS Plan, a plan for investment, a plan for reform*. The Stationery Office, London.

5 Campbell SM, Hann M, Hacker J *et al.* (2001) Identifying predictors of high quality care in English general practice: observational study. *BMJ*. **323**: 784.

Access

Services for patients

How many appointments are there available per patient per year?	Doctor(s)	Nurse(s)	Other team members
List size			
Total appointments			
Routine appointments			
Emergency appointments			
Total appointments per patient			
Routine appointments per patient			
Emergency appointments per patient			
Add up the **total time available** to patients and service users for consulting the team			
Separate this out between routine and emergency appointments			
Routine appointments			
Emergency appointments			
Total			

How many **appointment requests** are made each week? (Get the receptionists to keep a record of **the total number** of appointment requests made for each clinical professional for a full week)								

Does the number of appointments available **match the demand** (i.e. the number of requests)?								
No			Yes, just as long as there are plenty of 'emergency' appointments			Yes, easily. The practice is part of the Advanced Access programme and routinely checks to ensure capacity matches demand		
Score 1	Score 2	Score 3	Score 4	Score 5	Score 6	Score 7	Score 8	Score 9

What is the **current wait** for an appointment?

Doctor(s) G MBA FBA								
More than 10 surgeries			Fewer than 10 surgeries but more than 4 (MBA criteria = within 10 of the candidates' surgeries)			4 or fewer surgeries		
Score 1	Score 2	Score 3	Score 4	Score 5	Score 6	Score 7	Score 8	Score 9

Nurse(s)								
More than 10 surgeries			Fewer than 10 surgeries but more than 4			4 or fewer surgeries		
Score 1	Score 2	Score 3	Score 4	Score 5	Score 6	Score 7	Score 8	Score 9

Other **team members**	More than 10 surgeries			Fewer than 10 surgeries but more than 4			4 or fewer surgeries		
	Score 1	Score 2	Score 3	Score 4	Score 5	Score 6	Score 7	Score 8	Score 9
G When was **the wait** for a routine appointment last **audited**?	Never			More than a year ago			Regularly audited		
	Score 1	Score 2	Score 3	Score 4	Score 5	Score 6	Score 7	Score 8	Score 9
Repeat the process at three monthly intervals to assess whether this is changing									

Comments and notes:

The practice appointment system

(assess the appointments book)

		Score 1	Score 2	Score 3	Score 4	Score 5	Score 6	Score 7	Score 8	Score 9
ToS	Is each doctor available in line with his or her contractual obligations? PMS doctors may have different contractual arrangements. Randomly select eight weeks out of the last six months and calculate the average availability									
	Full-time (26 hours per week)?	Rarely			Most of the time			Yes all of the time		
	Three-quarters-time (19 hours per week)?	Rarely			Most of the time			Yes all of the time		
	Half-time (13 hours per week)?	Rarely			Most of the time			Yes all of the time		
ToS E QTD	Is the practice open during the **published opening hours** in the practice leaflet?	Rarely			Most of the time			Yes all of the time		

Comments and notes:

Routine appointments

E	Range of Appointment times:	Score 1	Score 2	Score 3	Score 4	Score 5	Score 6	Score 7	Score 8	Score 9
ToS	How many appointments does the practice offer **outside 9.00am–5.00pm?**	None or very few per week			One to five per day per team member consulting			More than five per day per team member consulting. The practice makes a genuine effort to provide a service to those who work or are unable to attend during the normal working day. The team members who provide services in unsocial hours are rewarded appropriately or given time off at other times		
QTD	What is the **booked length of each appointment?**	< 7.5 minutes			= 7.5 minutes			10 minutes (Quality[5])		
QTD QPA MAP FBA	What is the **actual average length of each consultation** (face to face)? (Most computerised appointment systems record this; alternatively, a stopwatch can be used to measure it. Record the length of consultations for a full week's worth of appointments, and work out the average)	< 5 minutes			5 to 7.5 minutes (MAP and FBA criteria)			> 7.5 minutes (Quality)		

G	How does the practice respond to an 'unacceptable' **wait for a *routine* appointment?**	Never audited so doctor(s) don't know!			Audited but rarely make appropriate changes			Respond by altering timetables and employing locums or assistants according to need (MAP and FBA)		
		Score 1	Score 2	Score 3	Score 4	Score 5	Score 6	Score 7	Score 8	Score 9
	What is the **wait for a *named* doctor?**	> 5 working days			2–5 working days			< 48 hours		
		Score 1	Score 2	Score 3	Score 4	Score 5	Score 6	Score 7	Score 8	Score 9

Comments and notes:

Emergency appointments

	Question	Scores 1–3	Scores 4–6	Scores 7–9
E	Does the practice have a written policy, available for patients and staff to see, for dealing with patients requesting an **emergency or same-day appointment?**	No, just a verbal agreement between staff and doctor	Yes, but it is not easily accessible to staff or patients and not written in practice leaflet	Yes, it is clearly available to patients and staff, and adhered to. It is included in the patients' leaflet
		Score 1 / Score 2 / Score 3	Score 4 / Score 5 / Score 6	Score 7 / Score 8 / Score 9
E QTD	Can patients always access a doctor or nurse within **48 hours?** (Ask the receptionists for their views!)	Sometimes	Most of the time	Always, there is a comprehensive triage and assessment system by one of the *clinical* staff
		Score 1 / Score 2 / Score 3	Score 4 / Score 5 / Score 6	Score 7 / Score 8 / Score 9
QTD	How many **emergency appointments** are requested per day?	Never counted	Counted, but doesn't alter the way the practice provides access or services	Regularly audited and does alter the way the practice responds and provides access to clinical staff
		Score 1 / Score 2 / Score 3	Score 4 / Score 5 / Score 6	Score 7 / Score 8 / Score 9
	Has the practice **asked patients or service users** about how easy it is to get an emergency appointment?	Never	Yes, a long time ago!	Yes, and the result affected the way the practice allocates emergency appointments for those who feel they have an urgent problem Alternatively, the practice is part of the 'Advanced Access' programme and this is irrelevant
		Score 1 / Score 2 / Score 3	Score 4 / Score 5 / Score 6	Score 7 / Score 8 / Score 9

Telephone access and consultations

G	How many **telephone lines** are there coming into the practice?	Several, but only one is available to patients			Several, but at busy times they are blocked so that it is difficult to get a line out to make a phone call			Plenty, there is never any difficulty phoning in or out of the practice. This has been assessed by BT to confirm this is not a significant problem		
		Score 1	Score 2	Score 3	Score 4	Score 5	Score 6	Score 7	Score 8	Score 9
	How many **staff are available** to answer telephone calls at the busiest times of the week?	One or two even at the busiest times			Varies according to the time of day and depending on how busy the practice is, but is not generally monitored			Regularly monitored, the policy is that if the frontline staff are busy there are others available to help out		
		Score 1	Score 2	Score 3	Score 4	Score 5	Score 6	Score 7	Score 8	Score 9

The assessor should try phoning into the practice on Monday mornings between 9.00am and 11.00am to see how frequently the line is engaged or how long the phone rings before it is answered

Has the practice ever used BT or any other mechanism to monitor how many calls fail to get through at their busiest times?

Comments and notes:

Duty doctor rota (group practices or those sharing rotas)

ToS E	Is there a clearly drawn up **duty doctor rota** for every day of the week, accessible to all staff?	No	Score 1	Score 2	Score 3	Yes but isn't regularly updated so may be inaccurate at times	Score 4	Score 5	Score 6	Yes. It is constantly updated on a week-to-week basis (or even during the week if necessary) and is posted in an easily accessible place in the practice	Score 7	Score 8	Score 9
E	What mechanism does the practice use for **contacting the duty doctor?**	No direct link	Score 1	Score 2	Score 3	Pager	Score 4	Score 5	Score 6	Mobile phone	Score 7	Score 8	Score 9
						Score 6 or 9 depending on how user-friendly the system is							
G	What mechanism does the practice have for providing 'continuity of care' and **handover of emergency problems?**	Write in notes	Score 1	Score 2	Score 3	Write in the notes and discuss informally at next practice meeting	Score 4	Score 5	Score 6	There is a practice protocol, which ensures formal handover takes place, including cases referred from the out-of-hours service. Records are also kept in the patients records	Score 7	Score 8	Score 9

Comments and notes:

Visits

E		Score 1	Score 2	Score 3		Score 4	Score 5	Score 6		Score 7	Score 8	Score 9
What system does the practice have to record **visit requests**?	Written on note-paper and handed to the doctor at some point				Recorded in a dedicated book for the doctor(s) to review at the end of surgery				Recorded in a book or diary *with the time as well as the date* the request was taken recorded. The person who takes the message signs the entry			
How are **visit requests allocated** to the doctors? (The assessor should consider asking the receptionists how the system runs as a measure of its efficiency)	The receptionist decides who might be able to find time to do the visits, there is no formal system for allocation				There is a system that is run by the reception staff for fair and efficient allocation				There is a written protocol, which includes discussion between doctors to ensure continuity of care for patients as well as fair and efficient allocation			

What mechanism does the practice have to ensure the **follow-up of patients who have been visited?**	The doctor remembers to carry out a follow-up visit when he or she next passes the door		The follow-up time is recorded in the patient's records and the patient is encouraged to request another visit in due course		The mechanism for follow-up is part of the visit allocation protocol and is recorded in the visit diary to ensure the follow-up is carried out and continuity of care provided	
	Score 1	Score 2	Score 3	Score 4	Score 5	Score 6	Score 7	Score 8	Score 9

Comments and notes:

Out-of-hours arrangements

T	What system does the practice use for out-of-hours arrangements?								
	Own on-call								
	Delegated to Healthcall or other out-of-hours provider								
	Co-operative or joint on-call service with another practice								
	Is the system used advertised in a practice leaflet and in the surgery?	No			Yes, but little detail is given on how to use the service			Yes. Clear instructions on the appropriate use of the out-of-hours services and how the system works are also described	
		Score 1	Score 2	Score 3	Score 4	Score 5	Score 6	Score 7	Score 8	Score 9

What mechanism is in place to ensure 'continuity of care' and **handover of emergency problems from the on-call service** takes place?	Don't know			Fax or telephone answer machine message is left by the on-call service			Fax or telephone answer machine message is left by the on-call service and, when necessary, the patients concerned are contacted by a member of the team to ensure that the problem has been solved adequately and appropriately		
	Score 1	Score 2	Score 3	Score 4	Score 5	Score 6	Score 7	Score 8	Score 9

Comments and notes:

Access to and quality of other services

Minor surgery

		Score 1	Score 2	Score 3	Score 4	Score 5	Score 6	Score 7	Score 8	Score 9
G	Are members of the practice **listed** with the health authority or PCT to carry out minor surgery?	No			Yes, but minor surgery is not something that the practice undertakes routinely			Yes, a full range of minor surgery procedures can be carried out by at least one doctor. The doctor(s) regularly attend update courses to ensure skills are maintained. The service is fully advertised in the surgery		
E	Does the practice have a policy regarding **'informed consent'** for minor surgery procedures?	No			Yes, usually verbal consent is obtained but this is not always recorded			Yes, a very strict policy. Written consent is obtained for all procedures. In many cases there is a written leaflet about the procedure explaining how it is carried out, any potential problems that could occur and how to obtain advice should the patient experience untoward effects following the procedure		

		Score 1	Score 2	Score 3	Score 4	Score 5	Score 6	Score 7	Score 8	Score 9
E	Does the practice keep **records of procedures** carried out?	Yes, most of the time			Yes, all of the time, but these records are for reference only			Yes, for every procedure carried out. The details of any drugs given before or during the procedure with the batch number and expiry date is recorded. There is a standardised method of recording details so that audit of results can be carried out at a later date		
G	Does the practice audit or **monitor the outcome** of minor surgery procedures?	No			Sometimes			Yes, a regular cycle of audit is carried out to monitor the rate of complications (for example, wound infections, the adequacy of post-surgical analgesia) and the overall outcome		

Does the practice have a policy of sending all **excised skin lesions to the pathology department** for histological examination?	No, only suspicious lesions are sent			Yes, all excised skin lesions are sent to the laboratory			Yes, all excised skin lesions are sent to the laboratory, and the audit process measures the rate of malignancies picked up and compares this with the level of suspicion of the surgeon at the time of excision		
	Score 1	Score 2	Score 3	Score 4	Score 5	Score 6	Score 7	Score 8	Score 9

Comments and notes

Child health and obstetric services
(other women's health issues are covered in Chapter 6)

G	Are members of the practice on the health authority's **child health surveillance list?**	No			Yes, but child health surveillance is not carried out by the practice			Yes, a full range of child health services and clinics are carried out by the practice		
		Score 1	Score 2	Score 3	Score 4	Score 5	Score 6	Score 7	Score 8	Score 9
	Does the practice run a multidisciplinary **child health service?**	No, the practice has difficulties getting other team members involved			Yes, the health visitors run the child surveillance clinics with doctor back-up. There are communication breakdowns at times, which could be improved			This is a true multidisciplinary service. Each team member has experience and qualifications in child health and there are good links to the paediatric hospital department, social services and other services including the voluntary sector. Communication between team members is generally very good. The whole team, including social workers, meet regularly to discuss specific cases as well as have educational meetings. The team has also sought input from service users		
		Score 1	Score 2	Score 3	Score 4	Score 5	Score 6	Score 7	Score 8	Score 9

		Score 1	Score 2	Score 3	Score 4	Score 5	Score 6	Score 7	Score 8	Score 9
G	Are members of the practice on the **health authority's obstetric list?**	No			Yes, but no protected time is set aside for maternity services. All maternity services are run within the routine surgeries and the midwife is rarely available at the time of seeing antenatal or postnatal women			Yes and a full range of maternity services, including intrapartum care, are provided. The practice runs specific maternity clinics at which the midwife and other key team personnel are available for consultation if necessary. The practice is equipped with all the necessary equipment including a modern Doppler foetal heart recording device. All team members ensure that their maternity skills are kept up to date		

Does the practice follow the UKCC midwifery antenatal screening guidelines?	No, the practice has no specific guidelines for provision of antenatal care		Yes, the guidelines are followed, but not audited or reviewed			Yes, the guidelines are not only adhered to but the midwife regularly updates the team on developments in midwifery and antenatal care. The care provided to pregnant women has been audited to ensure that all team members are following the guidelines. The notes are recorded in a standardised form to enable auditing (for example using a computer-based template)		
	Score 1	Score 2	Score 3	Score 4	Score 5	Score 6	Score 7	Score 8	Score 9

QTD	Does the practice promote **breastfeeding**?	No, not specifically. Practice members can offer advice if necessary			Yes, this is part of the routine antenatal education programme			Yes, there are trained breastfeeding counsellors who run specific classes for women during their antenatal period and they are available after delivery The practice audits its breastfeeding rates		
		Score 1	Score 2	Score 3	Score 4	Score 5	Score 6	Score 7	Score 8	Score 9

Comments and notes:

Other members of the primary healthcare team
(communication between team members is dealt with in Chapter 5)

G	Can patients access the other **members of the PHCT** through the practice?	No			Yes			Yes, this is clearly advertised in the surgery and in the practice leaflet.		
		Score 1	Score 2	Score 3	Score 4	Score 5	Score 6	Score 7	Score 8	Score 9

Access for those with disabilities

L	How easily can patients with **physical disabilities** gain access?	The surgery is not designed to allow easy access for those with anything other than minimal disability	There are access ramps and disabled facilities in and around the surgery, but improvements need to be made	The surgery was designed or modified with the disabled in mind. Doorways are all wide enough to allow wheelchair access; the facilities are all easily accessible for those with mobility problems. We actively encourage the use of the surgery by the disabled by ensuring there are grab rails and different types of chair in the waiting room to cater for those with different disabilities
		Score 1 Score 2 Score 3	Score 4 Score 5 Score 6	Score 7 Score 8 Score 9
	How are the needs of those with **visual impairments** met?	There are no special signs or facilities and/or the building really is not suitable for those with visual impairment	The building has suitable signs and consideration has been made, but the practice has not consulted visually impaired patients for further advice	The building has suitable signs and the different areas of the surgery are colour-coded and coordinated in such a way as to make movement around the building as easy as possible. The practice has consulted visually impaired patients for further advice. Staff are trained to look out for those with visual impairment to ensure that they are helped when necessary
		Score 1 Score 2 Score 3	Score 4 Score 5 Score 6	Score 7 Score 8 Score 9

G	Are the practice leaflet and other information leaflets available in large font sizes and **Braille**?	No			Yes, but these are available in English only. There is room for improvement in this area			Yes, they are available in large fonts and Braille as well as different languages. Staff are willing to read out the leaflets for those with visual impairment. The practice has consulted widely on this issue		
		Score 1	Score 2	Score 3	Score 4	Score 5	Score 6	Score 7	Score 8	Score 9
	How are the needs of those with **hearing difficulties** met?	No special consideration is made			The practice has special facilities for those with hearing difficulties. These include induction loops, but the practice has not consulted patients about making further improvements			The practice has extensive facilities including induction loops and minicom, and also has easy access to someone who can sign. The practice has consulted patients with hearing difficulties about making improvements		
		Score 1	Score 2	Score 3	Score 4	Score 5	Score 6	Score 7	Score 8	Score 9

G	Has the practice **consulted users** with various disabilities about special arrangements in the surgery?	No			Yes, but the practice was unable to implement suggestions			Yes, significant changes have been made to ensure that users with disabilities are catered for appropriately. Ongoing dialogue ensures that the practice continues to develop services and facilities for all users with disabilities		
		Score 1	Score 2	Score 3	Score 4	Score 5	Score 6	Score 7	Score 8	Score 9

Comments and notes:

Access for those who do not speak English

	Score 1	Score 2	Score 3	Score 4	Score 5	Score 6	Score 7	Score 8	Score 9
Does the practice have access to **interpreting services**? (This is covered in more detail in Chapter 5.)	No			Yes, but rarely used. The practice does not make special arrangements to run clinics with qualified interpreters available			Yes, the practice has access to authority-run services. The practice runs clinics specially organised with a fully qualified interpreter available throughout the clinic. Some staff speak other languages, but the practice is aware that using staff as interpreters can lead to difficulties, such as staff having their own prejudices which interfere with consultations. Further staff may be put in a difficult position regarding confidentiality. Therefore, staff are only used in emergency situations		

Comments and notes:

Access to notes and records

		Score 1	Score 2	Score 3	Score 4	Score 5	Score 6	Score 7	Score 8	Score 9
L	How easily can patients get **access to their records**?	We do not encourage access to records			Patients can ask to see their notes and an appointment is made for the patient to discuss the request with a doctor			We advertise that it is a patient's right to be able to have access to their records under the Data Protection Act (1999) and we have a leaflet explaining how a patient might get access to their records and any costs involved		
L	How easily can patients **access insurance (or other) medical reports?**	The report is kept for the obligatory 6 months and then destroyed			The report is kept on file and made available to the patient on request			The practice advertises that patients are entitled to see all medical reports before they are sent to the requester and make a positive effort to contact those patients that indicate that they wish to see the report to tell them that the report is written		

Total score, count the number of criteria scoring 1 and place the total in the first box, then the number scoring 2 and place in the second box and continue with scores 3, 4, 5, 6, 7, 8 and 9	The areas scoring 1, 2 or 3 **urgently** need to be put in place or need significant improvement			The areas scoring 4, 5 or 6 need reviewing and improving			The areas which are working well score 7, 8 or 9. Can the principles of these systems be transferred to other areas of practice work?		
Total scores	Score 1	Score 2	Score 3	Score 4	Score 5	Score 6	Score 7	Score 8	Score 9

L = legal requirement
G = considered good practice
MAP = Membership of the RCGP by Assessment of Performance

ToS = contractual or in Terms of Service
QTD = Quality Team Development

E = essential for revalidation
QPA = Quality Practice Award
FBA = Fellowship of the RCGP by Assessment of Performance

5

Building, environment and equipment

Background

> A doctor shall –
>
> (a) provide proper and sufficient accommodation at his practice premises, having regard to the circumstances of his practice; and
> (b) on receipt of a written request from the FHSA, allow inspection of those premises at a reasonable time by a member or officer of the FHSA or Local Medical Committee or both, authorised by the FHSA for the purpose.
>
> Paragraph 27 of the Terms of Service, of the National Health Service
> (General Medical Services) Regulations 1992

There must be as many definitions of 'proper and sufficient accommodation' as there are GP premises. They range from the most modern and well-equipped, state-of-the-art purpose-built buildings to barely converted high street shops or houses in residential roads. The key question is, are they 'fit for purpose'?

The GMC document *Good Medical Practice* clearly lays out the responsibilities that doctors have with regard to allowing patients comfort, dignity and privacy. There are many laws and statutory acts pertaining to the premises and equipment, all ensuring safety and access for patients and staff. These include: the Disability Discrimination Act of 1995 (DDA, 1995); the Health and Safety at Work Act (1974) and the associated COSHH regulations, which have many aspects of infection control within them; Health Service guidance on sterilisation equipment; and amendments to the GMS Regulations pertaining to the necessary room and equipment to carry out minor surgery in practice.

The Statement of Fees and Allowances (the 'Red Book') gives precise space allocations for reimbursement for cost-rent purposes. It is likely that most modern buildings have been constructed with these in mind, in order that doctors can work from the most spacious premises possible at no extra cost to themselves.

If practices want to carry out procedures over and above the prescribed minor surgery list, found in Schedule 6 of the NHS (General Medical Services) Regulations 1992, then they have to be registered as a nursing home, where the stipulations for buildings and equipment requirements are even stricter. Procedures carried out, such as sigmoidoscopies, would be included on the list as a procedure requiring registration as a nursing home.

All of the quality initiatives for general practice assess the building, environment and the equipment used by GPs in their surgeries. It is inevitable, therefore, that the process of revalidation of doctors will take into account these factors also.

The RCGP quality criteria take into account the structure and equipment of the surgery. It is expected that each professional consulting will have the appropriate equipment available. For doctors and nurses this includes stethoscope, sphygmo-manometer, thermometer, scales, height measure, peak flow meters (adult and child reading), otoscope and ophthalmoscope, tendon hammer and Snellen chart. It is not uncommon for me to be unable to find any evidence of a tendon hammer or height measure in consulting rooms! Locums also complain that they can't find basic equipment in even the best surgeries.

The practice 'face'

It is rare to find an underperforming practice working from good premises. The practice premises are the 'face' of the practice. The front door is usually the first aspect of the practice experienced by visitors, followed by the entrance hall and reception desk. If these are welcoming, clean and tidy, and well sign-posted, then the rest of the experience within the practice is likely to be positive. Unfortunately, the converse of this can be true also.

When was the last time you sat in the waiting room and actually looked at the environment in which patients frequently spend a considerable amount of time? The questions in this chapter explore the suitability of the practice environment from a patient's perspective, not forgetting those with disabilities.

It is interesting to note that in a Department of Health building visited by the author, the disabled toilets had all the usual wheelchair access and grab rails to assist wheelchair users in the lavatory, but the design of the basins and their height was such that no wheelchair user would ever be able to wash his or her hands!

Many GPs own their premises. Others rent from a private landlord; some work from premises owned by the health authority or primary care organisations (PCOs). For those GPs who retain their independent contractor status and own their own buildings, the conditions of their premises fall fairly and squarely on their own shoulders; for those renting or working in premises owned by others, the responsibility of the GP is to ensure that the owners keep the premises in a state of repair which falls within the law and provides the appropriate level of privacy and security which those using general practice in the 21st century expect.

Certainly, irrespective of owner, the cleanliness of the patient areas, in particular the clinical areas, is the responsibility of the GP or GPs working there. There is little excuse for dirty premises. Similarly, this is the case for the safety of staff and security of records and equipment.

Cleanliness and equipment maintenance

Patient safety within the surgery environment has to be paramount. The cleanliness of the building and the equipment are part of providing an environment that is safe for patients, especially if they are undergoing invasive procedures.

Vaccine fridges should be well maintained and records of regular temperature recordings kept. The purpose of this is to ensure that vaccines are kept at an optimal temperature to ensure they are effective when given. Most vaccines are easily rendered useless by being stored too warm or too cold. The optimal temperature for storage is usually recorded within the packaging. Of course, fridges should be regularly disinfected.

Likewise, sterilisation equipment should be regularly maintained and records of services should be kept. The importance of keeping such records would become very obvious if you were to be sued for the failure of a drug or vaccine previously kept in the fridge or for causing a significant wound infection.

Most practices have a service contract with a reputable engineer to service and maintain equipment on a regular basis, but not all.

During one assessment of a practice I carried out, I was given the treatment area as a base from which to work: a good opportunity to really assess the practice standards of infection control.

The vaccines fridge was a standard domestic fridge. The defrost plug at the back of the fridge was blocked. As such, the water generated on the defrosting plate passed down to the floor of the fridge where it collected in a sizeable puddle. The puddle reached such proportions at times that it ran out of the fridge door on to the floor of the treatment room, where it was collected by a dirty rag kept on the floor under the door.

In the puddle on the floor of the fridge was stored the current, in-date flu vaccine! Two shelves above the flu vaccine there was an uncovered piece of chocolate cake and a pot of coleslaw, well out of date. This food remained in the fridge for the full two weeks of the assessment. Also in the same fridge, were shelf after shelf of drugs and vaccines as much as four years out of date.

There was no evidence of a fridge thermometer and no records of the fridge temperature.

Security

Unfortunately, practice premises are vulnerable to break-ins. It is obvious that they will not only contain valuable computer equipment and other office equipment, but also are likely to have drugs on site.

It is now common place, particularly in inner cities, to see practices with metal shutters or grills over the windows to prevent forced entry. Despite the risks, I did assess a practice in London that didn't even have a burglar alarm. It is a requirement of the Quality Team Development programme of the RCGP.

Permanent external lighting can be a deterrent to casual burglars. The crime prevention officer at the local police station will be very willing to come and discuss all aspects of security of the surgery premises.

Staff deserve some level of security also. On two occasions I have been asked about how to deal with pilfering. It is always difficult to understand how in the close community of a surgery staff, one member (or more) can steal from their colleagues. One practice had such a problem they had to fit closed circuit monitoring, which showed the reception desk, to discourage the culprit. The difficulty is when the senior practice staff are fairly convinced they know who the culprit is, but are unable to prove it. One solution is to provide lockers for staff to store their belongings.

Furthermore, to ensure the security of money handed over the reception desk, all cash taken should be recorded and secured immediately, but this is, of course, cumbersome and surprisingly time-consuming at a busy reception desk.

It is not the place of this book to deal with serious fraud at a higher level, but there are well-documented cases of senior staff stealing from the practice by fraudulent means.

Violence against staff

Another aspect of security is preventing violence against staff. Since a survey carried out in September 1998, the government has taken this issue very seriously. This survey was carried out in 402 NHS trusts in England. It showed that approximately 65 000 violent incidents occur each year. The cost to the employee, in terms of physical or psychological pain, and stress, can be enormous. The costs to the NHS in terms of lost time at work, cost of temporary staff, legal action and counselling are also very considerable. This survey did not take into account those incidents occurring in general practice, but it is well recorded that they are not rare.

Practices have very different views about preventing violence or protecting staff. Some practices feel that an open-plan reception layout tends to make all patients and service users more comfortable and, therefore, less likely to become aggressive or violent. Others feel that staff should be protected and that glass shields should be in place. The argument here is that this type of barrier leads to feelings of animosity and, therefore, may even provoke aggressive behaviour. Clearly there are no right answers.

The Crime and Disorder Act (1998) stipulates that local authorities and police, in cooperation with other bodies including the NHS, are legally required to formulate and implement crime and disorder strategies. Health authorities should, therefore, have strategies and advice available to practices regarding violence towards staff. Many health authorities have arrangements with either police stations or walk-in centres to allow patients who are known to be violent to be seen on their premises. In practice, such arrangements are rarely used.

There is a lot of very useful information regarding this issue on the NHS website, www.nhs.uk/zerotolerance. There is a specific section aimed at primary care entitled, 'Primary care – preventing violence and abuse against general practitioners and their staff'. There is a booklet available to go with this section, which can be ordered on the website, but the health authority or primary care organisation should have copies. The website sets out the legal requirements of practices and useful advice about training staff in methods of recognising potentially aggressive or violent situations and preventing them from escalating. It also discusses the use of panic alarms and regular training on their use.

Once again, consult the crime prevention officer at the local police about preventing violence and also about self-defence.

Privacy, dignity and confidentiality

Basic patient care starts with the premise that confidentiality, privacy and dignity will be preserved at all times. Many lay people think that GPs believe this is a fallacy, especially when they have experiences like overhearing reception staff discussing patients. There are many things practices can do to improve the environment to ensure the maximum possible privacy, dignity and confidentiality.

Chapter 10 on staff management highlights the importance of training staff from the moment they start working in the practice about the principles of confidentiality. The staff contract should contain confidentiality clauses and these should be regularly reiterated. Certain aspects of receptionists' work can be carried out away from the reception area and this reduces the amount of discussion that needs to take place in front of people sitting in the waiting room. Staff training should also include ways of dealing with patients at the reception desk so that sensitive questions can be asked in discreet ways.

Soundproofing of surgery doors and walls should be part of the basic design; unfortunately this is not always the case. If the soundproofing is inadequate, then simple procedures like ensuring patients are not sitting next to consulting rooms during surgeries reduces the possibility that others will be party to the consultation taking place.

Privacy and dignity seem so fundamentally obvious, yet doctors do forget these issues. The author has assessed several practices where there are no curtains around the examination couch or no curtains at the windows, allowing full view of patients during consultations. I have also assessed practices where there were no curtains at the windows as well as no curtain around the couch; in one case the main ramp into the surgery ran past the window.

When this type of situation is pointed out to the doctor, replies like 'I have known my patients for so long they don't mind undressing in front of me' are the complacent excuse. Fortunately these are unusual, but serve to make the point about how easy it is to forget the fundamental rights of patients.

Safety

Providing a safe environment for staff usually means that the environment is safe for patients. Aspects of the Health and Safety at Work Act 1974 are covered in the questions in Chapter 9. The safety of patients and staff within the environment of the surgery is paramount. Questions in this section seek to explore whether aspects of safety have been taken into account.

In many cases, safety is common sense: not placing the kettle on the sink, close enough that staff can fill it without first unplugging it; not having the kettle on the floor; training staff to use potentially dangerous equipment (like paper shredders); ensuring fire exits are kept clear, are a few examples.

For patient safety, ensuring that fires or heaters are well guarded seems obvious, but ensuring that there isn't a pile of useful, but highly flammable, literature stored on top of the guard may not be so obvious to some.

The local council environmental health department runs basic courses in health and safety. Sending one or two members of staff along may be a sound investment. The fundamental lesson learnt is how to carry out a risk assessment, thereby ensuring an awareness of safety issues and preventing unnecessary accidents or fires.

The local fire station will offer advice about fire safety and prevention.

Basic amenities

The cleanliness and tidiness of the waiting room is discussed at the beginning of this chapter. Patients also have to use other amenities in the surgery, like the surgery toilet. Once again, the facilities available are a good measure of the quality of the respect for patients and the overall service provided. When did you last visit the patients' toilet at the surgery? Again, consider whether it is suitable for the disabled.

Premises improvements

Progressively over the past 10 to 15 years, the premises from which GPs practise have generally improved. The cost-rent scheme has enabled many doctors to purchase buildings with appropriate levels of reimbursement. The availability of improvement grants should have ensured that most doctors' surgeries are 'fit for purpose'.

Recently, the government has reviewed the quality of GP premises. A pan-London review of premises has provided information about the state of premises in the London area, and the Local Implementation Finance Trust (LIFT) scheme should ensure further improvements.

Other aspects of access to surgeries are dealt with in Chapter 4. It deals more directly with access for service users with disabilities and aspects of the Disability Discrimination Act 1995, directly affecting GPs, much of which will become legally binding in 2002.

I recently assessed a surgery that was a small shop in a high street. The waiting room was the front room of the shop. The windows were boarded up to within 12 inches of the top – allowing very little natural light in, but preventing those walking up the high street from seeing who was sitting in the waiting room.

The doctor's consulting room not only contained all the patients' files in filing cabinets, but it had no windows at all. There was just about room for the desk and examination couch.

The nurse's room was a back room of the shop. It was heated only by a bottled-gas heater, which filled the room with fumes. It was also the only access down into the basement, where the practice manager worked. Descending the extremely old wooden staircase was dangerous to say the least. There was vegetation growing out from the walls down the staircase.

Needless to say, the first task was to set a project in motion to get the practice to move to refurbished premises.

Key questions

- Are the practice premises 'fit for purpose'?
- Do the premises reflect an attitude of respect for all patients and users of the practice?
- Do the practice premises encourage access and use by disabled patients?

Building, environment and equipment

Surgery environment

ToS									
Are all the rooms in the surgery **warm and well lit**?	The waiting room is frequently cold in winter			Yes, but could be improved			Yes, all rooms, especially clinical rooms, are warm and appropriately lit to allow adequate examination		
	Score 1	Score 2	Score 3	Score 4	Score 5	Score 6	Score 7	Score 8	Score 9
Is the **waiting room** pleasant to sit in?	No, it is frequently cold in winter; it is in need of redecoration; it is invariably untidy. The posters and information leaflets are out of date. The magazines are very old			Yes, but could be improved. It is in need of redecorating but is kept clean and tidy. An effort is made to keep magazines, posters and leaflets up to date			Yes. The practice is fully aware that some patients spend a considerable amount of time in the waiting room and providing a pleasant environment reduces complaints about waiting times and has a bearing on the consultation to follow. It is also used as an educational environment for adults and children		
	Score 1	Score 2	Score 3	Score 4	Score 5	Score 6	Score 7	Score 8	Score 9

Question	Score 1	Score 2	Score 3	Score 4	Score 5	Score 6	Score 7	Score 8	Score 9
Is the waiting room **clean and tidy**?	No			Yes, but it is in need of redecoration, and the furniture is generally tatty			Yes, the décor is pleasant, cheerful and well maintained. The practice understands that some patients and users will need to sit for a significant amount of time in the waiting areas and it is essential that they are kept comfortable during that time, in order that the experience is as stress-free as possible		
How easy is it to **manoeuvre prams and pushchairs** in the surgery?	Generally difficult, with steps and narrow doorways to negotiate			It is possible without too much difficulty, but there is nowhere for them to be safely left			The design of the building took this into account, and the gangways and doorways are wide and easily negotiated. There is an area dedicated to parking prams and pushchairs, which is as secure as it can be		

		Score 1	Score 2	Score 3	Score 4	Score 5	Score 6	Score 7	Score 8	Score 9
G	Are there **toys for children** to play with in the waiting room?	No, or those that are there are old and broken; as such they are dangerous. They have been stolen in the past and have not been replaced			Yes, but they are generally sparse and not in very good condition			Yes, the practice is aware that children who are unoccupied become fractious and uncooperative. This upsets the parent or carer and has an adverse effect on the consultation. The waiting room is, therefore, a pleasant environment for children. The play area is slightly separate from the main waiting room to avoid unnecessary noise for those patients wishing to sit quietly		
E	Can **patients be overheard** while talking to the reception staff, by people sitting in the waiting room?	Yes, there are chairs in the waiting room that are very close to the reception desk. Most conversations can be overheard			Sometimes. The receptionists are aware of this problem and are careful to keep this to a minimum			No. The reception desk and waiting room layout was specially designed with this issue in mind, and it is very difficult to overhear conversations. This is also the case with telephone conversations between patients and reception staff		

		Score 1	Score 2	Score 3	Score 4	Score 5	Score 6	Score 7	Score 8	Score 9
L	How easily can patients with **physical disabilities** gain access?	The surgery is not designed to allow easy access for those with anything other than minimal disability			There are access ramps and disabled facilities in and around the surgery but improvements need to be made			The surgery was designed or modified with the disabled in mind. Doorways are all wide enough to allow wheelchair access, the facilities are all easily accessible for those with sensory and mobility problems. The practice actively encourages the use of the surgery by those with a disability		
L	Is the practice aware of the fact that since October 1999 aspects of **Disability Discrimination Act 1995** (DDA) are legally binding and they are open to legal action if they don't comply?	No. The practice was unaware of this Act and does not encourage patients with disabilities at all			Yes, but the practice has done little to discover how this might affect the surgery			Yes. The practice has consulted a local disability organisation as well as service users with disabilities about the surgery and has started planning changes to make the environment far more accessible for service users with all kinds of disabilities		

	Score 1	Score 2	Score 3	Score 4	Score 5	Score 6	Score 7	Score 8	Score 9
Is the **patients' toilet** warm and clean?	No. It is old, not regularly cleaned. It has become an unpleasant environment and there is no hot water running to the basin. Towels are not provided to dry hands on after washing them			Yes, but is in need of redecoration. There is plenty of hot and cold water running to the basin and the towels are clean (or paper towels are provided)			Yes, it is cleaned regularly, sometimes more than once in a day if necessary. It is warm. There is plenty of hot and cold running water and towels are clean (or paper towels always in plentiful supply). There are baby changing facilities as well		
	Score 1	Score 2	Score 3	Score 4	Score 5	Score 6	Score 7	Score 8	Score 9
Is the toilet designed for those in **wheelchairs**?	No, it is only accessible by walking up or down stairs			Yes, but manoeuvring a wheelchair would be very difficult. The hand basin would be difficult to reach from a wheelchair			Yes, the whole building design incorporated ideas to help those with disabilities, irrespective of their disability. Local disability organisations were consulted about developments and design		
	Score 1	Score 2	Score 3	Score 4	Score 5	Score 6	Score 7	Score 8	Score 9

Comments and notes:

Privacy and dignity

		Score 1	Score 2	Score 3	Score 4	Score 5	Score 6	Score 7	Score 8	Score 9
E	Do all rooms have a sheet or a **blanket** so that patients can cover themselves to retain dignity while being examined?	No, some do not			Yes, but there are occasions when it is not used			Yes, there is an ongoing programme to ensure that the patients' right to privacy and dignity is understood and remembered at all times		
E	Do all consulting rooms have either windows designed, or are there **curtains or blinds** at the windows, so that people cannot see in from outside?	No, this has not been considered before			Yes, but the curtains are not always drawn			Yes, the design is such that total privacy and dignity can be maintained at all times. If this is not the case, staff are regularly warned that curtains must be closed when consulting		

E	Does every consulting room have access to an **examination couch** and each couch have a curtain round it for patients to dress and undress in privacy?	No			Yes, but there is no ongoing check to ensure that clinical staff are fully aware of the issue of patient privacy and dignity. It is very much assumed that clinical staff are aware that they should preserve patients' dignity			Yes, privacy, dignity and confidentiality are regularly discussed at meetings with all staff		
		Score 1	Score 2	Score 3	Score 4	Score 5	Score 6	Score 7	Score 8	Score 9

Comments and notes:

Security

E	Does the **reception desk** provide a secure and safe environment for the staff?	No, this has not been considered or there is a security grill of some kind at the reception desk			Yes, this was considered in the initial design, but there are still examples where patients are aggressive towards the staff. Further assessment and changes to the reception area, for example, are necessary			Yes, great consideration was taken into account during the design of the surgery. The practice has a good balance between staff safety and patient acceptability. Advice has been listened to		
		Score 1	Score 2	Score 3	Score 4	Score 5	Score 6	Score 7	Score 8	Score 9
	Does the practice have **adequate security**?	No, there are no burglar or panic alarms. There have been break-ins and violence towards staff in the past and these measures were still not put in place			Barely adequate precautions are in place. There have been break-ins, and no security advice was sought after these. Panic alarms do exist in some rooms including the reception area, but there is no policy or training about when or how to use them			Yes. There have been no break-ins for a long time. The security system was recently updated. The system is regularly serviced and checked. Staff are instructed about exactly how and when to use the systems available		
		Score 1	Score 2	Score 3	Score 4	Score 5	Score 6	Score 7	Score 8	Score 9

Comments and notes:

Equipment

Does the practice have the following **equipment available** to each doctor and nurse or other attached staff member in each consulting room – remember the rooms used by locums or temporary staff?

	Place a tick in the appropriate box	
	No	Yes
1 Stethoscope		
2 Sphygmomanometer		
3 Scales		
4 Height chart		
5 Peak flow meter (child)		
6 Peak flow meter (adult)		
7 Tape measure		
8 Tendon hammer		
9 Otoscope		
10 Ophthalmoscope		
11 Snellen chart		

Count up the ticks in the 'yes' column and score accordingly	Fewer than 5 items Score 1	5 items Score 2	6 items Score 3	7 items Score 4	8 items Score 5	9 items Score 6	10 items Score 7	11 only Score 8	All 11 items or more Score 9

QTD	**Sphygmomanometers** When were the sphygmomanometers last calibrated?	Don't know, or don't think they ever have been			At least 12 months ago			Within 12 months. There is a system of getting either a pharmaceutical company or the local hospital to calibrate sphygmomanometers every year (or more frequently)		
		Score 1	Score 2	Score 3	Score 4	Score 5	Score 6	Score 7	Score 8	Score 9

If the practice has a branch surgery, all the above questions should be answered for the branch surgery as well

Comments and notes:

	Score 1	Score 2	Score 3	Score 4	Score 5	Score 6	Score 7	Score 8	Score 9
Does the practice have a policy of **maintaining or upgrading equipment** on a regular basis?	No, maintenance rarely occurs and equipment is generally old and outdated. There are no contingency plans in place for equipment replacement and this occurs as a last resort			Yes, equipment is repaired when necessary and new equipment is purchased when it is deemed unsafe or legislation changes which forces replacement. Records of maintenance and replacement are not kept			Yes. The practice budgets for maintenance and replacement. The practice is aware that legislation changes mean that equipment becomes obsolete. Each member of staff who uses a piece of equipment is responsible for notifying the practice manager or one of the doctors if equipment is faulty or due for replacement, so that a decision to replace the item can be made before a crisis occurs		

Electrical equipment

		Score 1	Score 2	Score 3	Score 4	Score 5	Score 6	Score 7	Score 8	Score 9
E	Does the practice have a **service contract** with an electrical engineer to check functioning and safety of the electrical equipment on a regular basis? This includes equipment like nebulisers and ECG machines	No, the electrical equipment has not been serviced or checked since purchase or for a long time			No, there is no service contract but the equipment is serviced irregularly. Records of services are kept			Yes, there is a service contract and services are carried out on a regular basis. The autoclave and other sterilisation equipment is checked every three months. Other equipment is checked on advice of the maintenance company. Full records are kept		
L	**Autoclave** Does the practice autoclave have the facility to do audit trails of equipment placed in it?	No, the practice wasn't aware that this is necessary			No, but audit trails are kept manually and there are plans to purchase appropriate equipment in the future			Yes. Alternatively, practices may use a Central Sterilise Supply Department (CSSD) at a local hospital instead of doing the sterilisation themselves. This is probably the best solution for practices carrying out considerable amounts of minor surgery or invasive procedures		

L	**Vaccines fridge** Is the vaccines fridge a commercially available fridge specially designed for the storage of vaccines, with an externally read temperature gauge?	No, it is a domestic fridge. There is no thermometer (or there is a thermometer but it is rarely read). Records of the internal temperature are not kept			No, but the fridge temperature is carefully monitored and the contents insured against fridge failure. The fridge temperature is read twice daily and records of the readings are kept			Yes, and there is a constant readout of the internal temperature of the fridge. This record is kept		
		Score 1	Score 2	Score 3	Score 4	Score 5	Score 6	Score 7	Score 8	Score 9
	When were the **contents of the fridge** last audited?	Never or a long time ago (can't remember!). The contents of the fridge are assessed once in a while and discarded if out of date			Within 12 months. At that time many drugs and vaccines were out of date and discarded. There is no policy to ensure routine review of the fridge contents but the practice nurse does it when necessary			Within the last six months. There is a log of all the fridge contents, clearly showing when replacement is necessary. There is a member of staff who has responsibility to ensure that the fridge contents, especially the vaccines, are kept up to date. It is the responsibility of each doctor to ensure that the contents of their medical bags are kept up to date and a recent audit showed that 90% of the drugs in doctors' bags were in date – the rest were changed immediately!		
		Score 1	Score 2	Score 3	Score 4	Score 5	Score 6	Score 7	Score 8	Score 9

Total score, count the number of criteria scoring 1 and place the total in the first box, then the number scoring 2 and place in the second box and continue with scores 3, 4, 5, 6, 7, 8 and 9	The areas scoring 1, 2 or 3 **urgently** need to be put in place or need significant improvement			The areas scoring 4, 5 or 6 need reviewing and improving			The areas which are working well score 7, 8 or 9. Can the principles of these systems be transferred to other areas of practice work?		
Total scores	Score 1	Score 2	Score 3	Score 4	Score 5	Score 6	Score 7	Score 8	Score 9

L = legal requirement
G = considered good practice
MAP = Membership of the RCGP by Assessment of Performance
ToS = contractual or in Terms of Service
QTD = Quality Team Development
E = essential for revalidation
QPA = Quality Practice Award
FBA = Fellowship of the RCGP by Assessment of Performance

PART TWO
PATIENT MANAGEMENT AND TREATMENT

Extreme remedies are most appropriate for extreme diseases.

Hippocrates 460–357 BC

6

Health promotion and chronic disease management

Background

In 1992, the NHS (GMS) Regulations for GPs were changed to include health promotion activities. Some of these were statutory. Not all attracted additional payment and with some that did it was no longer a straightforward item of service payment as before, but dependent on hitting targets set by the government.

These activities included:

- GPs having to offer an annual assessment to all those on the list aged 75 or over (Schedule 2, Terms of Service for doctors, paragraph 16). The prescribed aspects of the assessment are listed later in this chapter.
- Controversial payment for childhood vaccinations and cervical screening was made on attainment of hitting prescribed targets.
- Payment for doctors carrying out a consultation with newly registered patients on the list (Part VI paragraph 14, (2) (l)). Once again, a prescribed list of questions and examination to be undertaken was listed in the regulations, and is included later in this chapter.
- Payment for doctors who register with the health authority and provide child health surveillance (Part VI paragraph 14, (2) (m)).
- Inducements to provide 'health promotion clinics approved by the FHSA' (Part VI paragraph 14, (2) (p)).

In the Government's White Paper *Saving Lives: our healthier nation,*[1] published in 1999, the NHS has been charged with reducing 'untimely and unnecessary deaths'. This White Paper set out ambitious targets to be reached by 2010, to reduce mortality from the main killers: cancer, coronary heart disease and stroke, accidents and mental illness.

There can be very few PHCTs that haven't been focusing for many years now on childhood vaccination programmes, screening for certain cancers, primarily cervical cancer, and screening for hypertension, as well as running other health promotion clinics.

Surely, it is the quality of the health promotional activities along with the management of chronic diseases that are the hallmarks of the overall quality of practice service delivery. Campbell *et al.*[2] used the chronic disease management of asthma, diabetes and angina as part of an assessment of the variation in the quality of care delivered by general practices. Interestingly, this study indicated that:

> No single type of practice has a monopoly on high quality care – small practices provide better access but poorer diabetes care.

Clinical governance

Both health promotion and chronic disease management cover every aspect of clinical governance. They incorporate aspects of team working and, therefore, communication. They often involve a much wider team than just the PHCT: attached staff, podiatrists, dieticians, hospital departments and social service departments are frequently involved in the overall care of patients with ongoing illness. Most practices develop policies and protocols for running health promotion clinics and it is vital that they apply 'evidence-based medicine' in their treatment of those with chronic diseases. This, therefore, requires that a development and review programme of the 'evidence-based guidelines' or protocols be in place.

A regular programme of continuing medical education (CME) for the whole team needs to feed into this process and this can be a good example of where practice needs and team members' personal development needs can be combined, as discussed in Chapter 10.

Good health promotion and chronic disease management rely heavily on recall systems, accurate disease registers, and policies for handling and recording results of investigations, as well as accurate record keeping. Monitoring the service provided is vital in order to maintain or improve it. This monitoring or audit is made very much easier if patients' records of chronic disease management are computerised.

Audits carried out by the author during practice assessments have shown that, in certain areas, diabetic patients are seen irregularly by the local hospital and at the most annually. From the letters returned to the practice, it appears that the monitoring is in no way standardised or thorough. Obviously, this will vary from area to area, but it is an indication that primary care has the key responsibility for chronic disease management. Further, assessment of chronic disease management is a good way of evaluating continuity of care within a practice.

Quality assessments

The RCGP quality criteria focus on health promotion and chronic disease management as well. Quality Team Development, for example, expects the team to identify:

> ... the health needs of their population, deliver appropriate preventive health services, and work[s] with their patients, other agencies and their community to promote health.

The college also expects practices to have developed protocols for asthma, diabetes, hypertension, coronary heart disease and 'at least one other'.

Protocols and guidelines

There are many of these available to 'take off the shelf', but the process of developing them or adapting those already available by the practice is very useful for educational purposes. It usually means that there is a 'champion for the cause' among the team and this enhances the care offered still further.

Protocols should contain built-in monitoring or audit processes, such as audit of adherence to the protocol. The protocol should also include the standards of service that the practice expects to reach, so that this can be compared with the actual level attained. Ultimately, practices should audit 'patient outcomes', but if based on evidence, then outcomes should improve.

Recall systems

To achieve vaccination and cervical smear targets, practices need robust, reliable recall systems. In the author's experience, practices that run their own recall systems have the highest immunisation and cervical smear rates. Delegating the recall systems to enthusiastic staff is the most efficient and successful way of encouraging patients to take up the service.

The recall systems have to be backed up by policies which ensure that those patients who fail to respond to letters offering services are followed up.

Clinical audit

Paragraph 7 of *Good Medical Practice* (GMC) is explicit in its expectation of doctors that they must take part in regular medical and clinical audit and, where necessary, respond to the results of audit to improve practice. Further, doctors must respond constructively to assessments and appraisals of professional competence.

In *Good Medical Practice for General Practitioners*,[3] there is a clear explanation of the implications of this statement by the GMC. It sets out how the 'excellent' GP reviews his or her knowledge and performance using a range of methods to monitor different aspects of care. Further, he or she uses these to develop practice and personal development plans.

The whole clinical governance agenda is underpinned by audit. Certainly the CHI sees it as one of the seven 'pillars' of clinical governance. CHI clinical governance reviews of NHS organisations include a review of the management and practice of clinical audit programmes.

GPs must, therefore, engage in the process of audit or other methods of monitoring the care they are offering. An assessment of practices, therefore, should include audit programmes.

The questions in this chapter focus on whether the practice uses evidence-based protocols and guidelines; who are the main users of these; the practice recall systems and other aspects of health promotion and chronic disease management. It also contains questions related to clinical audit.

Key questions

- Does the practice have a genuine commitment to promote the health of its patients and service users, and to provide comprehensive chronic disease management?
- Is it clear who has responsibility to ensure uptake of services and follow-up of non-responders?
- Are the services and outcomes monitored?

References

1 Department of Health (1999) *Saving Lives: our healthier nation*. The Stationery Office, London.

2 Campbell SM, Hann M, Hacker J *et al.* (2001) Identifying predictors of high quality general practice; observational study. *BMJ*. **323**: 784–7.

3 General Practitioners Committee and Royal College of General Practitioners (2000) *Good Medical Practice for General Practitioners*. GPC and RCGP, London.

Health promotion, chronic disease management

Health promotion

	What target levels does the practice achieve?	(Missed)			(Lower rate)			(Higher rate) QTD, MAP and FBA	
E	**Cervical smears** 50% (lower rate) and 80% (higher rate) (ages 25–64)	< 30% Score 1	30–39% Score 2	41–49% Score 3	50–59% Score 4	60–69% Score 5	70–79% Score 6	80–89% Score 8	> 90% Score 9
	Childhood immunisations								
	70% (lower rate) 90% (higher rate) *Under 2*			< 50% Score 1	50–59% Score 2	60–69% Score 3	70–79% Score 5	80–89% Score 7	> 90% Score 9
E	DTP, 3 doses								
E	Pertussis, 3 doses								
E	MMR, 3 doses								
E	Pre-school boosters								

Women's health

		Score 1	Score 2	Score 3	Score 4	Score 5	Score 6	Score 7	Score 8	Score 9
G	Does the practice run its own **cervical smear recall system?**	No, the practice relies solely on the health authority system			Yes, when the health authority system fails to get patients to attend for smears			Yes, the practice has a dedicated member of staff who runs the system on a month-by-month rolling programme		
QTD	Does the practice have policy to **follow up those who fail to turn up?**	No, the health authority system will send another reminder in due course			Yes, the practice undertakes to write to the patient			The practice not only writes to the patient, but also labels the records so that the failure to attend can be discussed at the next routine appointment. The dedicated member of staff has a clear protocol on how to deal with non-responders, and this includes a policy to bring this to the attention of the patient's registered doctor after failure to attend after a set number of reminders		
		Score 1	Score 2	Score 3	Score 4	Score 5	Score 6	Score 7	Score 8	Score 9

	Score 1	Score 2	Score 3	Score 4	Score 5	Score 6	Score 7	Score 8	Score 9
E QTD — Does the practice have a written policy for informing women of their **smear results**? Is a summary of these instructions given to women at the time of taking the smear?	No, but women are asked or expected to phone in for their results			Yes, there is a written policy that sets out that all women with *abnormal results* are contacted about their results, but those with normal results are expected to phone the practice			Yes there is a written policy that sets out that all women are written to, informing them of the result, normal or abnormal. An information sheet explaining this is given to women after they have had a smear. Further information about the next smear or what to do if they have a question about their smear, is included		
G QTD — Does the practice **audit its smear quality**?	No, occasionally the practice receives notification about this from the health authority. No action is taken			Yes, it is noted but no action is taken as a result of this			Yes, if the rate of 'inadequate quality' starts rising, specific retraining is considered and arranged if necessary		
G — Does the practice **monitor smear results** to ensure that all those women with abnormal smears are re-smeared or seen at the hospital with pre-determined and agreed deadlines?	No			Yes, but not regularly. Little or no action was taken last time the audit was undertaken			A regular audit cycle is undertaken and the recall system and the results are discussed with the hospital if necessary		

Other services for women
(antenatal services are discussed in Chapter 4)

QTD		Score 1	Score 2	Score 3	Score 4	Score 5	Score 6	Score 7	Score 8	Score 9
	Does the practice provide **family planning and sexual health** services?	No, contraception is available at a family planning clinic held elsewhere			Yes, the service runs as part of the routine surgeries, it does not provide cap and coil-fitting services			Yes, the practice runs a comprehensive service providing oral contraceptive advice as well as cap and coil fitting. The personnel running the service regularly attend update courses and educate the other team members also		
E	Does the practice have a policy to ensure that young women have adequate **protection against rubella**?	No			Yes, it is mentioned as part of the routine discussion on contraception			Yes, as well as being mentioned as part of the routine discussion on contraception, we actively promote measurement of rubella antibody titres, followed by immunisation if titres are inadequate. This service is advertised in the waiting room, in the practice leaflet and in clinical rooms. There is a separate leaflet given to young women when they attend the surgery for whatever reason		
		Score 1	Score 2	Score 3	Score 4	Score 5	Score 6	Score 7	Score 8	Score 9

G	Does the practice have a policy to 'fast track' women who need **emergency contraception?**								
	No, they are sent to the family planning clinic			Yes, they are tagged on the end of emergency surgeries. In order to be seen, they have to explain to the receptionist the nature of the problem			Yes, there is a policy in which all staff are trained. This ensures that these women are seen with minimal explanation and are immediately directed to one of the contraceptive-trained personnel. The practice consulted a local women's group and/or a teenage group to seek their advice about the best way to offer a comprehensive, safe, confidential service for this group		
	Score 1	Score 2	Score 3	Score 4	Score 5	Score 6	Score 7	Score 8	Score 9

Does the practice dedicate time to **promote women's health?**	No, but women are offered advice about their health in routine surgeries		Yes, a specifically trained member of the team runs a 'Well Woman' clinic				Yes, a specifically trained member of the team runs a clinic. The team member regularly attends update courses and educates the rest of the team if appropriate. Women and local women's groups were consulted about the running of the clinic before the protocols were written and the clinic was set up. It is regularly audited to ensure that the service provided is acceptable and worthwhile for those attending, and also to ensure that the clinic protocols are followed. There are good links with other members of the PHCT and even links outside the team, for example to social services		
	Score 1	Score 2	Score 3	Score 4	Score 5	Score 6	Score 7	Score 8	Score 9

| QTD | Does the practice have a policy to encourage women to attend for **breast screening**? | No | Score 1 | Score 2 | Score 3 | Score 4 | Yes, the practice team members discuss this in routine surgeries, particularly when women ask for advice about hormone replacement therapy | Score 5 | Score 6 | Yes, the practice constantly monitors uptake of the service and ensures that non-responders are chased. The records of non-responders are tagged so that breast screening can be discussed at subsequent surgery attendances. Women are invited to discuss breast screening when we are aware that they are approaching an appointment for screening. There are posters about breast screening in the surgery, and it is mentioned in the practice leaflet | Score 7 | Score 8 | Score 9 |
| | Does the practice have a policy for dealing with **domestic violence**? | No | Score 1 | Score 2 | Score 3 | Score 4 | No, but one is planned and the team is aware and has discussed the issues | Score 5 | Score 6 | Yes, this policy ensures all team members are aware of the issues and know where to go to get help for those subjected to domestic violence. The policy had input from local women's groups, a women's refuge, the police and victim support unit, and/or the probation service | Score 7 | Score 8 | Score 9 |

Child health services

Is the practice listed to provide **child health surveillance?**	No			Yes, one partner is (or more partners are) listed but have not been to update courses for several years			Yes, one or more partners are listed. They regularly update their knowledge. One partner in particular is a child health specialist and is used as a 'consultant' within the practice		
	Score 1	Score 2	Score 3	Score 4	Score 5	Score 6	Score 7	Score 8	Score 9
E Does the practice run its own **vaccination and immunisation recall system?**	The practice uses the health authority system			Yes, but it is used mainly when the practice fails to reach its immunisation targets			Yes. The practice has a dedicated member of staff who runs the system, in conjunction with the health visitors, on a month-by-month rolling programme		
	Score 1	Score 2	Score 3	Score 4	Score 5	Score 6	Score 7	Score 8	Score 9

		Score 1	Score 2	Score 3	Score 4	Score 5	Score 6	Score 7	Score 8	Score 9
G	Does the practice have a written policy about how to follow-up those **families who fail to turn up for immunisation?**	No			No written policy, but the families are discussed between the team. It is the responsibility of the health visitor to follow up non-responders. The practice undertakes to write to the patient if necessary			Yes. The policy sets out that not only does the person in charge of the vaccination recall system write to the patient, but also informs the health visitors of the non-responders. Further, the records are marked so that the failure to be immunised can be discussed at the next routine appointment. The policy ensures that persistent non-responders are brought to the attention of the registered doctor so that further action can be taken		
	Is the practice fully aware of the law surrounding **child protection** issues?	Not adequately			Yes, but the practice does need updating			Yes. The practice is fully aware of the Children's Act and their responsibilities to attend case conferences. One partner has responsibility to keep the whole practice up to date in child protection issues. There are good links with social services and the probation service		

Men's health

		Score 1	Score 2	Score 3	Score 4	Score 5	Score 6	Score 7	Score 8	Score 9
G	Does the practice dedicate time to promote **'men's health'**?	No			No, but there is a lot of promotional literature in the surgery persuading men of the importance of exercise, healthy diet and regular review of blood pressure and urinalysis. Further, there is information available about testicular cancer			Yes. One team member is specifically qualified in 'men's health' and runs dedicated clinics. The team member ensures that he or she attends regular update courses and acts as a 'consultant' for other team members. The issues are regularly discussed in team meetings. The clinic is audited for attendance and outcomes		
ToS	Does the practice have a policy and procedure for inviting those patients (aged between 16 and 75) **not seen for 3 years**, to attend 'for the purpose of assessing whether' there are any health needs?	No			Yes, but this is not a high priority and is not done very regularly			Yes, this is done regularly. The practice sees this as an integral part of health promotion activities, and as a mechanism for offering services to those who are less likely to attend but may have health needs		

New patient assessments

ToS	Does the practice regularly offer assessment to **new patients** joining the list?	No or yes, but attendance is necessary before the patient is allowed to join the list			Yes, but uptake is very patchy and the practice does not follow up non-attendees			Yes. This is seen as a very good way to screen new patients, get to know them and to ensure that they are aware of the services offered by the practice. Uptake is over 85%		
		Score 1	Score 2	Score 3	Score 4	Score 5	Score 6	Score 7	Score 8	Score 9
								No (or don't know)	Yes	
ToS	Does the **new patient assessment** contain the following *history:* (Place ticks in the appropriate columns)									
1	Details of patient's medical history									
2	Family history									
3	Hereditary conditions									
4	Immunisation history									
5	Allergies									
6	Medication									
7	Tests carried out for breast or cervical cancer									
8	Social factors (including housing, employment and family circumstances)									
9	Lifestyle (including diet, exercise, smoking and alcohol consumption, misuse of drugs)									
10	Current state of health									
Count the number of ticks in the 'Yes' column		No ticks Score 1	1 tick Score 2	2 ticks Score 3	3 ticks Score 4	4 ticks Score 5	5 ticks Score 6	6 ticks Score 7	7 ticks Score 8	> 8 ticks Score 9

ToS	Does the **new patient assessment** contain the following *examination*: (Place ticks in the appropriate columns)	No (or don't know)	Yes
1	Measurement of height		
2	Weight		
3	Blood pressure		
4	Urine for		
	(a) Protein		
	(b) Glucose		

Count the number of ticks in the 'Yes' column	No ticks Score 1	1 tick Score 2	2 ticks Score 3	3 ticks Score 4	4 ticks Score 6	5 ticks Score 7	5 ticks and more items examined Score 9

Comments and notes:

Over-75 annual reviews

ToS	Does the practice have a protocol for offering patients **over 75 years of age an annual health assessment?**	No			Yes, the district nurses run this with minimal input from the doctors		Yes. This is seen as a team responsibility. It fits in with the annual flu vaccination programme. Patients not taking up the service are telephoned to ensure that there are no obvious health needs. It is a service that is audited carefully to follow uptake and ensure that the team members adhere to the guidelines and protocol
		Score 1	Score 2	Score 3	Score 4	Score 5	Score 6	Score 7	Score 8	Score 9

ToS	Does the **over-75 assessment** contain the following: (Place ticks in the appropriate columns)	No (or don't know)	Yes
1	Sensory functions		
2	Mobility		
3	Mental condition		
4	Physical condition		
	(a) Continence		
	(b) Urinary protein		
	(c) Urinary glucose		
	(d) Presence of haematuria		
	(e) Weight		
	(f) Blood pressure		
5	Social environment		
6	Use of medicines		
	Count the number of ticks in the 'Yes' column		

< 5 ticks Score 1	5 ticks Score 2	6 ticks Score 3	7 ticks Score 4	8 ticks Score 5	9 ticks Score 6	10 ticks Score 7	11 ticks Score 8	11 ticks and more assessed Score 9

Chronic disease management
Coronary heart disease

QTD	Does the practice dedicate time for **specific health promotional activities**, which includes patients with coronary heart disease (CHD)?	No, all care of those with CHD is carried out as part of the routine surgery			Yes, a clinic is run by the nurse with little input from other team members			Yes, it is seen as an essential way in which patients with CHD are properly monitored and cared for. It is truly multidisciplinary with close links to outside agencies including the hospital department. Patients have had an input into the running of the clinic		
		Score 1	Score 2	Score 3	Score 4	Score 5	Score 6	Score 7	Score 8	Score 9
QTD	Is there a written **evidence-based protocol** for managing patients with CHD?	No			Yes, but it has not been reviewed for over two years			Yes, it is reviewed annually, or updated if a team member goes on an update course and shows that further developments can be included in the protocol. The protocol is clear about responsibilities and accountabilities. It is clear in the protocol when patients with complications should be referred to the hospital; this has been agreed with the hospital department		
		Score 1	Score 2	Score 3	Score 4	Score 5	Score 6	Score 7	Score 8	Score 9

	Score 1	Score 2	Score 3	Score 4	Score 5	Score 6	Score 7	Score 8	Score 9
Is there a **lead person**, ensuring that the protocol is adhered to?	No			Yes, the practice nurse			Yes, the team member is valued as offering not only a unique service to the patients, but also a key educational resource for the whole team. The lead person is the key link to the outside agencies and ensures the smooth running of the clinic		
Is there a specified person responsible for the **recall system**?	No, patients are expected to attend the surgery when their medication review date comes up			Yes, it is the nurse or whoever runs the clinic			Yes. This person supports the lead person and ensures that the lead person is fully aware of patients who fail to turn up to clinics and who may need encouragement to attend. They also have responsibility for ensuring that patients requiring hospital support get this appropriately. They may also be aware when patients are admitted to hospital for further intervention		

Does the practice regularly **monitor** the service provided?	No				Yes, the clinic has been audited but this is not done regularly		Yes, the protocol has a built-in mechanism to ensure audit is carried out regularly. The results are discussed at practice meetings and changes to the clinic made if necessary. The audit measures adherence to the protocol and outcomes, like the control of blood pressure, cholesterol levels and the rate of complications		
	Score 1	Score 2	Score 3	Score 4	Score 5	Score 6	Score 7	Score 8	Score 9

Hypertension

	Score 1	Score 2	Score 3	Score 4	Score 5	Score 6	Score 7	Score 8	Score 9
Does the practice dedicate time for **specific health promotional activities**, which includes patients with hypertension?	No, all care of those with hypertension is carried out as part of the routine surgery			Yes, a clinic is run by the nurse with little input from other team members			Yes, it is seen as an essential way in which patients with hypertension are properly monitored and cared for. It is owned and run by the whole practice and not just the responsibility of one person. Patients have had an input into the running of the clinic		
Is there a written **evidence-based protocol** managing patients with hypertension?	No			Yes, but it has not been reviewed for over two years.			Yes, it is reviewed annually or updated if a team member goes on an update course and shows that further developments can be included in the protocol. The protocol is clear about responsibilities and accountabilities. It is clear in the protocol when patients with complications or poor blood pressure control should be referred to the hospital; this has been agreed with the hospital department		
	Score 1	Score 2	Score 3	Score 4	Score 5	Score 6	Score 7	Score 8	Score 9

	Score 1	Score 2	Score 3	Score 4	Score 5	Score 6	Score 7	Score 8	Score 9
Is there a **lead person** for running the clinic and ensuring that the protocol is adhered to?	No			Yes, the practice nurse			Yes, the team member is valued as offering not only a unique service to the patients, but also a key educational resource for the whole team. The lead person is the key link to the outside agencies and ensures the smooth running of the clinic		
Is there a specified person responsible for the **recall system**?	No, patients are expected to attend the surgery when their medication review date comes up			Yes, it is the nurse or whoever runs the clinic			Yes, this person supports the lead person and ensures that the lead person is fully aware of patients who fail to turn up to clinics and who may need encouragement to attend. They also have responsibility for ensuring that patients requiring hospital support get this appropriately. They may also be aware when patients are admitted to hospital for complications or other reasons (e.g. stroke)		

Does the practice regularly **monitor** the service provided?	No			Yes, the clinic has been audited but this is not done regularly			Yes, the protocol has a built-in mechanism to ensure audit is carried out regularly. The results are discussed at practice meetings and changes to the clinic made if necessary. The audit measures adherence to the protocol and outcomes, like the control of blood pressure, monitoring of renal function and blood electrolytes, especially for those on medication		
	Score 1	Score 2	Score 3	Score 4	Score 5	Score 6	Score 7	Score 8	Score 9

Stroke

QTD									
Does the practice dedicate time for **specific health promotional activities**, which includes patients with stroke?	No, all care following a stroke is carried out as part of the routine surgery			Yes, a clinic is run by the nurse with little input from other team members			Yes, it is seen as an essential way in which patients who have had a stroke are properly monitored and cared for. It is truly multidisciplinary with close links to outside agencies including the hospital department and social services. Patients and their carers have had an input into the running of the clinic		
	Score 1	Score 2	Score 3	Score 4	Score 5	Score 6	Score 7	Score 8	Score 9
Does the practice **offer support to those caring** for patients severely disabled by their stroke?	No			This is done by an outside agency			Yes, there are information packs given to the carer on how to make contact with each member of the team, including the attached staff, and other agencies like social services. The practice makes a point of including carers in all decisions made about the patient, as seems appropriate		
	Score 1	Score 2	Score 3	Score 4	Score 5	Score 6	Score 7	Score 8	Score 9

	Score 1	Score 2	Score 3	Score 4	Score 5	Score 6	Score 7	Score 8	Score 9
Does the practice ensure that **homebound** stroke victims are visited regularly?	No			Yes, this is done by the district nurse or a doctor. It rarely involves other team members			Yes, this is a multidisciplinary team function with a key worker who ensures that a regular needs assessment is made and the appropriate team members informed that further input is needed. This is seen as proactive management and enhances the care of the patient and supports the carer. Regular team meetings assist in this process		
QTD Is there a **written evidence-based protocol** for the management of acute stroke as well as the ongoing care of stroke patients?	No			Yes, but it has not been reviewed for over two years			Yes, it is reviewed annually or updated if a team member goes on an update course and shows that further developments can be included in the protocol. The protocol is clear about responsibilities and accountabilities. It is clear in the protocol when patients with complications like deterioration in function or mobility should be referred to the appropriate hospital department; this has been agreed with the hospital department		

	Score 1	Score 2	Score 3	Score 4	Score 5	Score 6	Score 7	Score 8	Score 9
Is there a **lead person** for running the clinic and ensuring that the protocol is adhered to?	No			Yes, the practice nurse			Yes, the team member is valued as offering not only a unique service to the patients, but also a key educational resource for the whole team. The lead person is the key link to the outside agencies and ensures the smooth running of the clinic		
Is there a specified person responsible for the **recall** system for those patients well enough to attend the clinic?	No, patients are expected to attend the surgery when their medication review date comes up			Yes, it is the nurse or whoever runs the clinic			Yes, this person supports the lead person (or is the lead person) and ensures that the lead person is fully aware of patients who fail to turn up to clinics and who may need encouragement to attend. They also have responsibility for ensuring that patients requiring hospital support get this appropriately. They may also be aware when patients are admitted to hospital for further intervention or recurrence of their stroke		

Does the practice regularly **monitor** the care provided to stroke patients?	No	Yes, the clinic has been audited but this is not done regularly	Yes, the protocol has a built-in mechanism to ensure audit is carried out regularly. The results are discussed at practice meetings and changes to the clinic made if necessary. The audit measures adherence to the protocol, and outcomes, like the control of blood pressure, monitoring of function and mobility, and rate of recurrence of strokes
	Score 1	Score 2	Score 3	Score 4	Score 5	Score 6	Score 7	Score 8	Score 9

Diabetes

	Score 1	Score 2	Score 3	Score 4	Score 5	Score 6	Score 7	Score 8	Score 9
Does the practice dedicate time for **specific health promotional** activities, which includes patients with diabetes?	No, all care of those with diabetes is carried out as part of the routine surgery			Yes, a clinic is run by the nurse with little input from other team members			Yes, it is seen as an essential way in which patients with diabetes are properly monitored and cared for. It is truly multidisciplinary with close links to outside agencies including the hospital department. Patients have had an input into the running of the clinic		
Is there a written **evidence-based protocol** for the management of patients with diabetes?	No			Yes, but it has not been reviewed for over two years			Yes, it is reviewed annually or updated if a team member goes on an update course and shows that further developments can be included in the protocol. The protocol is clear about responsibilities and accountabilities. It is clear in the protocol when patients with complications should be referred to the hospital; this has been agreed with the hospital department		

	Score 1	Score 2	Score 3	Score 4	Score 5	Score 6	Score 7	Score 8	Score 9
Is there a **lead person** for running the clinic and ensuring that the diabetes protocol is adhered to?	No			Yes, the practice nurse			Yes, the team member is valued as offering not only a unique service to the patients, but also a key educational resource for the whole team. The lead person is the key link to the outside agencies and ensures the smooth running of the clinic		
Is there a specified person responsible for the **recall system** for those patients attending the clinic or ensuring that those that don't are monitored?	No, patients are expected to attend the surgery when their medication review date comes up			Yes, it the nurse or whoever runs the clinic			Yes, this person supports the lead person (or is the lead person) and ensures that the lead person is fully aware of patients who fail to turn up to clinics and who may need encouragement to attend. They also have responsibility for ensuring that patients requiring hospital support get this appropriately. They may also be aware when patients are admitted to hospital for further intervention		

Does the practice regularly **monitor** the care provided to diabetic patients?	No			Yes, the clinic has been audited but this is not done regularly			Yes, the protocol has a built-in mechanism to ensure audit is carried out regularly. The results are discussed at practice meetings and changes to the clinic made if necessary. The audit measures adherence to the protocol and outcomes, like the control of blood pressure, HbA1C levels, cholesterol levels, renal function and the rate of complications as well as admissions with acute hypo-glycaemic or hyperglycaemic and ketoacidotic episodes		
	Score 1	Score 2	Score 3	Score 4	Score 5	Score 6	Score 7	Score 8	Score 9

Asthma and chronic obstructive airways disease (COPD)

	Score 1	Score 2	Score 3	Score 4	Score 5	Score 6	Score 7	Score 8	Score 9
Does the practice dedicate time for **specific health promotional activities**, including those aimed at patients with asthma and COPD?	No, all care of those with asthma and COPD is carried out as part of the routine surgery			Yes, a clinic is run by the nurse with little input from other team members			Yes, it is seen as an essential way in which patients with asthma and COPD are properly monitored and cared for. It is truly multi-disciplinary with close links to outside agencies including the hospital department. Patients have had an input into the running of the clinic		
Is there a written **evidence-based protocol** for the management of those with asthma or COPD?	No			Yes, but it has not been reviewed for over two years			Yes, it is reviewed annually or updated if a team member goes on an update course and shows that further developments can be included in the protocol. The protocol is clear about responsibilities and accountabilities. It is clear in the protocol when patients with complications should be referred to the hospital; this has been agreed with the hospital department		

		Score 1	Score 2	Score 3	Score 4	Score 5	Score 6	Score 7	Score 8	Score 9
Is there a **lead person** for running the clinic and ensuring that the protocol is adhered to?	No				Yes, the practice nurse			Yes, the team member is valued as offering not only a unique service to the patients, but also a key educational resource for the whole team. The lead person is the key link to the outside agencies and ensures the smooth running of the clinic		
Is there a specified person responsible for the **recall system** ensuring that patients are reviewed and monitored regularly?	No, patients are expected to attend the surgery when their medication review date comes up				Yes, the nurse or whoever runs the clinic			Yes, this person supports the lead person (or is the lead person) and ensures that the lead person is fully aware of patients who fail to turn up to clinics and who may need encouragement to attend. They also have responsibility for ensuring that patients requiring hospital support get this appropriately. They may also be aware when patients are admitted to hospital with an acute exacerbation		

Does the practice regularly **monitor** the care provided to patients with asthma or COPD?	No	Yes, the clinic has been audited but this is not done regularly	Yes, the protocol has a built-in mechanism to ensure audit is carried out regularly. The results are discussed at practice meetings and changes to the clinic made if necessary. The audit measures adherence to the protocol and outcomes, like the control of peak flow, nocturnal coughing, growth and weight (of children), and the rate of admissions with acute exacerbations
	Score 1	Score 2	Score 3	Score 4	Score 5	Score 6	Score 7	Score 8	Score 9

Other chronic diseases specifically focused on by the practice

Does the practice run other **specific services for patients with chronic illness** not mentioned above?	No, all care of those with chronic illness is carried out as part of the routine surgery			Yes, clinics are run by the nurse with little input from other team members			Yes, dedicated time is seen as an essential way in which patients with chronic diseases are properly monitored and cared for. It is truly multidisciplinary with close links to outside agencies including the hospital department and other appropriate outside bodies. Patients have had an input into the running of the clinic
	Score 1	Score 2	Score 3	Score 4	Score 5	Score 6	Score 7 Score 8 Score 9
Are there other written **evidence-based protocols** for the management of the chronic illness?	No			Yes, but they have not been reviewed for over two years			Yes, they are reviewed annually or updated if a team member goes on an update course and shows that further developments can be included in the protocol. The protocol is clear about responsibilities and accountabilities. It is clear in the protocol when patients with complications should be referred to the hospital; this has been agreed with the hospital department
	Score 1	Score 2	Score 3	Score 4	Score 5	Score 6	Score 7 Score 8 Score 9

Question	Score 1	Score 2	Score 3	Score 4	Score 5	Score 6	Score 7	Score 8	Score 9
Is there a **lead person** for running of such clinics ensuring that the protocols are adhered to?	No			Yes, the practice nurse			Yes, the team member is valued as offering a unique service, not only to the patients but also as a key educational resource for the whole team. The lead person is the key link to the outside agencies and ensures the smooth running of the clinic		
Is there a **specified person** responsible for the recall system?	No, patients are expected to attend the surgery when their medication review date comes up			Yes, it the nurse or whoever runs the clinic			Yes, this person supports the lead person (or is the lead person) and ensures that the lead person is fully aware of patients who fail to turn up to clinics and who may need encouragement to attend. They also have responsibility for ensuring that patients requiring hospital support get this appropriately. They may also be aware when patients are admitted to hospital for further intervention		

	Score 1	Score 2	Score 3	Score 4	Score 5	Score 6	Score 7	Score 8	Score 9
Does the practice regularly **monitor** the care provided to these patients?	No			Yes, the clinic has been audited but this is not done regularly			Yes, the protocol has a built-in mechanism to ensure audit is carried out regularly. The results are discussed at practice meetings and changes to the clinic made if necessary. The audit measures adherence to the protocol and appropriate outcomes, like the rate of admissions with acute exacerbations		
	Score 1	Score 2	Score 3	Score 4	Score 5	Score 6	Score 7	Score 8	Score 9
Total score, count the number of criteria scoring 1 and place the total in the first box, then the number scoring 2 and place in the second box and continue with scores 3, 4, 5, 6, 7, 8 and 9	The areas scoring 1, 2 or 3 **urgently** need to be put in place or need significant improvement			The areas scoring 4, 5 or 6 need reviewing and improving			The areas which are working well score 7, 8 or 9. Can the principles of these systems be transferred to other areas of practice work?		
Total scores	Score 1	Score 2	Score 3	Score 4	Score 5	Score 6	Score 7	Score 8	Score 9

L = legal requirement
G = considered good practice
MAP = Membership of the RCGP by Assessment of Performance

ToS = contractual or in Terms of Service
QTD = Quality Team Development

E = essential for revalidation
QPA = Quality Practice Award
FBA = Fellowship of the RCGP by Assessment of Performance

7

Prescribing

Background

Few GPs can fail to understand the importance of sound prescribing policies. The supplement to the National Service Framework for Older People, *Medicines and Older People*,[1] cites some pretty appalling statistics about prescribing; for example, between 5 and 17% of hospital admissions are related to adverse drug reactions,[2] and 6 to 17% of older patients experience adverse drug reactions.[3,4]

Unpublished audits of repeat prescribing in London show that up to 20 scripts per day can be generated per GP, with patients taking as many as 13 separate drugs at any one time. This forms a large part of the practice workload and poses significant clinical governance issues for practices and primary care organisations.

> In one London practice of 2500 patients, the number of items on repeat prescriptions averaged 3.9 per patient (range 1 to 13). Thirty three per cent of patients requesting repeat prescriptions were taking five or more medications at once. In another practice, the average was seven (range 1 to 23) and 67% were taking five or more medications at once.
>
> This gives some idea of not only the workload but also the potential drug interactions. It emphasises the importance of regular medication reviews.

This chapter doesn't enter into the minefield of prescribing budgets and cost-effective prescribing. Inevitably, however, sound prescribing policies and an awareness of good practice in the field of prescribing do influence costs.

The GMC's document *Good Medical Practice* puts responsibility on every doctor to regard the efficacy of treatments and the use of resources prudently. On the other hand, doctors must prescribe treatment, drugs or appliances that meet the patient's needs. Section 6 of the GPC and RCGP document *Good Medical Practice for General Practitioners* elaborates how only effective treatments should be prescribed and that an 'unacceptable' GP prescribes ineffective treatments, takes no account of cost and refuses to register patients taking expensive treatments. Many health authorities use prescribing data from the Prescription Pricing Authority (PPA) as indicators of quality of service provision in primary care. These indicators are all controversial.

The RCGP includes prescribing and management policies of doctors and practices in its assessment for Membership and Fellowship of the college by assessment of performance.

This chapter questions some of the vital aspects of the practice prescribing policies which ensure patient safety and minimise the risks of prescribing.

Computer-based prescribing

Most practices now use computers for the production and recording of prescribing, both acute and repeat prescribing. Not all doctors use computers during consultations and, as such, the prescriptions written during consultations are not recorded in the patient's computerised records. The issues of inaccurate or incomplete records are discussed in Chapter 8.

The advantages of computer-based prescribing have been well documented. The *BMJ* editorial 'Computer based prescribing'[5] summarises them. In essence, computer-based prescribing has been shown to help doctors make better decisions by offering ranked lists of suitable drugs. The list is usually chosen from a locally agreed drug formulary. Computers should also highlight drug allergies and interactions.

Furthermore, computer tools have been shown to increase generic prescribing, improve legibility and, therefore, reduce pharmacy inquiries. It is claimed that they have also reduced costs,[5,6] both in terms of drug costs and staff time for writing repeat prescriptions.

Repeat prescribing

All practices should have a repeat prescribing policy which allows patients efficient, safe access to prescriptions for ongoing medications, but doesn't allow patients to abuse the system and hoard unnecessary drugs. The questions in this section assess the robust nature of the practice's repeat prescribing policy.

Key questions

- Is the practice aware of the importance of sound acute and repeat prescribing policies?
- Does the practice prescribe in line with evidence-based principles?
- Does the practice make a conscious effort to monitor prescribing habits?

References

1   Department of Health (2001) *Medicines and Older People*. The Stationery Office, London.

2   Cunningham G, Dodd TRP, Grant DJ *et al.* (1997) Drug related problems in elderly patients admitted to Tayside hospitals, methods for prevention and subsequent reassessment. *Age & Aging*. **26**: 375–82.

3   Mannesse CK, Derkx FH, de Ridder MA *et al.* (2000) Contribution of adverse drug reaction to hospital admission of older patients. *Age & Aging*. **29**: 35–9.

4   Mannesse CK, Derkx FH, de Ridder MA *et al.* (1997) Adverse drug reactions in elderly patients as a contributing factor for hospital admission: cross sectional study. *BMJ*. **315**: 1057–8.

5   Wyatt J, Walton R (1995) Computer based prescribing. *BMJ*. **311**: 1181–2.

6   Dowell JS, Snadden D, Dunbar JA (1995) Changing to generic formulary: how one fund-holding practice reduced prescribing costs. *BMJ*. **310**: 505–8.

Prescribing

	Score 1	Score 2	Score 3	Score 4	Score 5	Score 6	Score 7	Score 8	Score 9
QTD MAP — What is the practice **generic prescribing rate?** *Beware! A very high generic prescribing rate (above 85%) is probably not cost-effective and may indicate differences in prescribing habits which need discussion*	Less than 50%			50–65%			65–80%		
QTD MAP — Does the practice assess and use **PACT** (Prescribing Analyses and Cost) **or SPA** (Scottish Prescribing Analysis) **data** to evaluate their prescribing habits?	No			Yes, occasionally. The practice has never requested higher-level PACT or SPA data, for an in-depth assessment			Yes. The practice regularly discusses the PACT data as an educational tool as well as assessing cost-effectiveness of prescribing. Higher levels of PACT data were used to draw up the practice formulary		

Does the practice use any prescribing habits as a **measurement of performance**? For example: • salbutamol to inhaled steroid ratio • antibiotic prescribing rate • quinolone to routine antibiotic ratio • antidepressant prescribing habits (tricyclics: SSRIs)	No			Yes, this has been done but does not change prescribing habits			Yes. These and other performance measures of prescribing are regularly used and discussed among the team		
	Score 1	Score 2	Score 3	Score 4	Score 5	Score 6	Score 7	Score 8	Score 9
Does the practice use a computer for **repeat prescribing**?	No			Yes			Yes, it is also the mechanism by which patients are recalled for medication reviews		
	Score 1	Score 2	Score 3	Score 4	Score 5	Score 6	Score 7	Score 8	Score 9

	Score 1	Score 2	Score 3	Score 4	Score 5	Score 6	Score 7	Score 8	Score 9
Does the practice use the computer for **acute prescribing**?	No			Yes, most of the time. Some prescriptions written on home visits, for example, are not recorded on the computer			Yes, all of the time, even prescriptions issued on home visits are recorded		
QTD Does the practice have a locally agreed **drug formulary** that is used most of the time? (This information should be provided in the practice annual report for the health authority)	No			Yes, audit shows that it is adhered to at the following levels:			Yes, and the practice monitors the adherence. The following results are achieved:		
	Score 1	Score 2	Score 3	Score 4 40–49%	Score 5 50–59%	Score 6 60–69%	Score 7 70–79%	Score 8 80–89%	Score 9 90% +

Comments and notes:

Storage and administration of drugs

			Score 1	Score 2	Score 3	Score 4	Score 5	Score 6	Score 7	Score 8	Score 9
L	Is the practice aware of the **Consumer Protection (Product Liability) Act 1987?**	No				Yes, vaguely			Yes, the necessary guidance is filed where it is accessible. The practice holds records of the sources of all products purchased. Likewise the practice records to whom drugs or vaccines are dispensed or administered		
L	Are records of the **source of all stored drugs** kept in the surgery?	Frequently no record of the source of the drug is made. Sometimes patients return unwanted drugs and these are stored for use by another patient. (This is not only extremely bad practice, but it is indefensible in the event of a complaint against the doctor)				Most of the time a record of the source of drugs is made			A record of the source of every drug and vaccine is made and kept for many years. Drugs are never taken back from patients, unless they can be disposed of correctly		

		Score 1	Score 2	Score 3	Score 4	Score 5	Score 6	Score 7	Score 8	Score 9
L, E	**How are controlled drugs stored** and recorded in the surgery?	Kept in locked cupboard			Kept in secure, approved cupboard and irregularly recorded			Kept in secure, locked cupboard along with the DDA record, according to the Misuse of Drugs Regulations 1985 & 2000. Every time a controlled drug is administered it is properly recorded and replaced		
E	**Emergency drugs** Does the practice have a reasonable store of up-to-date emergency drugs available to all doctors?	Yes, but these are rarely checked as to whether they are still in date. No record of administration is made			Yes, they are available and regularly checked to ensure they are in date. Drugs are administered sometimes without a record being made			Yes, they are regularly checked to ensure they are in date, and there is a regular programme of education and courses to ensure all members of the team know how and when it is appropriate to use the drugs. Every time a drug is administered a record of the event is made in the patient's notes and a separate register of administration is also kept		

Comments and notes:

Repeat prescribing

QTD		Score 1	Score 2	Score 3		Score 4	Score 5	Score 6		Score 7	Score 8	Score 9
Does the practice have a *written* **repeat prescribing** policy?	No	Score 1	Score 2	Score 3	Yes, but it has not been audited or reviewed	Score 4	Score 5	Score 6	Yes, and it contains a commitment to regular review and audit	Score 7	Score 8	Score 9
Does the practice have a policy for **regularly reviewing** patients who take long-term medication?	Yes, but it is not written down	Score 1	Score 2	Score 3	Yes, it is part of the repeat prescribing policy, but has not been recently audited	Score 4	Score 5	Score 6	Yes. It is regularly audited to ensure 80% adherence, and was audited less than two years ago	Score 7	Score 8	Score 9
Who has **access** to the written policy?	We have no written policy	Score 1	Score 2	Score 3	Doctors only	Score 4	Score 5	Score 6	Everyone who needs access to the policy: • doctors • nurses • practice manager • staff involved in dealing with repeat prescriptions • local community pharmacist	Score 7	Score 8	Score 9

Question	Score 1	Score 2	Score 3	Score 4	Score 5	Score 6	Score 7	Score 8	Score 9
Do the practice staff have **specific training** in the handling of repeat prescriptions?	No			Yes			Yes, and they are regularly updated about changes to the policy, and given the opportunity to feed back about how well it works. Furthermore, they are appraised about repeat prescriptions to ensure that they adhere to the policy		
If the practice uses a **paper system** for recording repeat prescriptions, does it have a separate up-to-date repeat drug record card?	No, the drugs are recorded chronologically in the notes. It is not easy to see all the medication taken at one time			Yes, but the system easily gets out of date and the date for the next medication review is not recorded			Yes. Clear records are kept of the currently taken drugs, as well as the date that the next medication review is due		
Does the practice have a **computerised repeat prescription** process?	No			Yes, but it is not used all of the time. The repeat prescription screen is out of date at least 50% of the time (do an audit to assess how up to date the screen is)			Yes, it is used all of the time. The repeat prescription screen is kept fully up to date (at least 85% of the time)		
Does the practice use the computer system to remind staff that patients need a **medication review?**	No			Yes, but it easily gets out of date and is adhered to only about 60% of the time			Yes. Audit shows that it is kept up to date and adhered to at least 80% of the time		

Do patients *have* to use computer-generated **repeat prescription counterfoils** to order repeat prescriptions?	No			Yes, most of the time (40–70%)			Yes, all of the time, except in exceptional circumstances when very ill patients are unable to use the system		
	Score 1	Score 2	Score 3	Score 4	Score 5	Score 6	Score 7	Score 8	Score 9
How do patients *not* using computer-generated repeat prescription counterfoils request repeat medications? How are these requests: • recorded • monitored? Consider carrying out an audit of the frequency patients have their repeat medication monitored. Do not count routine or emergency appointments; only count genuine repeat medication monitoring appointments. Score the practice 1 to 9 according to how well the system works									
	Score 1	Score 2	Score 3	Score 4	Score 5	Score 6	Score 7	Score 8	Score 9

	Score 1	Score 2	Score 3	Score 4	Score 5	Score 6	Score 7	Score 8	Score 9
Does the repeat prescription policy clearly explain to the administrative staff when the doctor will require the **patients' notes**?	No			Yes, but still the notes are shown to the doctor unnecessarily or not when they should be			Yes, the policy is clear. The notes are always consulted when: • the patient takes more than four medications • the patient has not been seen within six months • the request does not match the computer record • the hospital (or another colleague) has altered a drug or dosage • the patient is particularly elderly or ill		
Has the practice **audited** the time it takes from when the patient makes the request to when the prescription is ready for collection?	No			Yes, it was over two working days for over 50% of requests and the system hasn't changed to improve this			Yes, it was within two working days for over 90% of requests. Alternatively, it was over two working days for about 60% of requests and the system has been changed to improve on this and the audit is about to be repeated		

	The areas scoring 1, 2 or 3 **urgently** need to be put in place or need significant improvement			The areas scoring 4, 5 or 6 need reviewing and improving			The areas which are working well score 7, 8 or 9. Can the principles of these systems be transferred to other areas of practice work?		
Total score, count the number of criteria scoring 1 and place the total in the first box, then the number scoring 2 and place in the second box and continue with scores 3, 4, 5, 6, 7, 8 and 9									
Total scores	Score 1	Score 2	Score 3	Score 4	Score 5	Score 6	Score 7	Score 8	Score 9

L = legal requirement
G = considered good practice
MAP = Membership of the RCGP by Assessment of Performance

ToS = contractual or in Terms of Service
QTD = Quality Team Development

E = essential for revalidation
QPA = Quality Practice Award
FBA = Fellowship of the RCGP by Assessment of Performance

8

Record keeping and letters

Background

Paragraph 36 of the Terms of Service, NHS (General Medical Services) Regulations 1992, makes keeping 'adequate records' a statutory obligation for GPs.

In *Good Medical Practice for GPs*,[1] the chapter on 'Keeping records and keeping your colleagues informed' comes immediately after the one entitled 'Good clinical care'. It sets out some very basic standards. These include paper records being legible and being entered in chronological order, along with reports and hospital letters being filed in date order. As with every chapter in *Good Medical Practice for GPs*, the section on notes and record keeping ends with examples of the standard of record keeping of the 'excellent GP' and that of the 'unacceptable GP'.

The RCGP, in all its quality criteria, highlights the importance of accurate, tidy note keeping and has very clear criteria necessary to achieve Membership and Fellowship of the college by assessment.

Those who have had to assess records for the purposes of advising health authority complaints departments will recognise the importance of clear, coherent and objective notes without subjective derogatory comments. It is very difficult to support a colleague who is being complained about if there are poor records of the event in question and the quality of note keeping is generally poor.

And, of course, medical indemnity companies repeatedly emphasise the necessity of good note keeping. A doctor's main defence comes from his or her records of the events that took place at the time in question.

For these reasons, many PCOs have, quite rightly, put quality of record keeping on their clinical governance agenda.

The 'paperless practice'

Electronic Patient Records (EPRs) and the concept of the 'paperless practice', with all the clinical governance issues surrounding these, are considered in Chapter 9.

Continuity of care

The completeness of records for continuity of care cannot be emphasised enough. Try asking a colleague to discuss the aspects of continuity of the care of a patient just from your notes. Immediately your colleague will consider whether the notes:

- contain a summary of significant past illnesses or on-going problems
- contain clear comprehensive entries of recent events
- clearly list whether the medications are taken on a long-term basis
- contain a list of drug allergies.

This is the most fundamental information necessary to treat a patient you have never seen before. If the practice uses locums or other temporary staff on a regular basis, these features should be glaringly obvious in the patients' records.

Letters from colleagues

Even the best practices have difficulty keeping up with the vast volume of letters that arrive on a daily basis. Once filing gets behind, it takes a disproportionate amount of time to catch up.

> The author assessed an excellent practice where the doctors were all clinically excellent, the practice manager very efficient and the building first class.
> Unfortunately, one doctor failed to return letters to be filed. The consulting room desk and floor were piled high with letters and the corresponding notes; some letters dated back over two years. Locums working in the practice complained that as many as a third of the notes for their surgeries were 'missing' and they were given a single new card to write on.

Practices do also face the problem of storage of vast mountains of paper coming into the practice. As such, many practices are now scanning letters on to their computer systems. The issues concerned with this are discussed in Chapter 12.

For those practices using EPRs but *not* scanning letters into the records, there remains a further problem. One clear reason for using the computer to store consultation records is to alleviate the time-consuming exercise of pulling patients' handwritten notes from storage shelves and returning them after surgeries. If the only place letters are stored is the handwritten record, then some records still need to be retrieved during the surgery. If the letters are all scanned on to the computer, then they are easily accessible at any time.

Letters to colleagues

The information contained in letters leaving the practice, for whatever purpose, is vitally important to the care of the patient. However, such communications are also a 'window' into the working of the practice. A tidy, well-formatted letter says a lot about the whole presentation of the practice, as does a poorly scribbled note.

GPs write letters for many reasons to all sorts of recipients. However, the majority of letters leaving the practice are referrals to hospital consultant colleagues. The clinical details within letters can directly affect patient care. The importance of the contents of letters to colleagues is, therefore, recognised in *Good Medical Practice for GPs* and in the Royal College criteria for Membership and Fellowship by Assessment.

First, most hospital consultants vet their referrals to decide the priority that should be given to the patient; the more information available, the easier the process of prioritisation. A GP's assessment of the urgency goes a long way towards assisting in the prioritisation process.

Second, if a consultant is given all the information regarding drugs taken, allergies and all the investigations carried out, this will frequently save time for the patient and NHS resources. Most referral letters should, therefore, contain:

- patient identification information
- clinical information
- other relevant information.

A detailed assessment of the quality of referral letters is suggested later in the chapter. Hopefully the practice of writing letters that read 'Please see and advise' has ended.

One practice recently assessed by the author had a template for referral letters that simply had to be completed by the referrer by hand. Several parts had tick boxes. Thus the handwritten letters were excellent quality and very quickly written.

Setting up a template on word processors is easily achieved, but the referrer does need to remember to dictate all the sections if the letter is completed by a secretary.

A letter received in a rheumatology department read:

Dear consultant,
This photographer who stands all day has a painful ankle. Please see and treat.
Thank you very much for seeing him.
Yours sincerely.

After the routine eight-month wait, the uncomplaining, 35-year-old photographer, with a family to support, hobbled into the department with a very swollen, inflamed ankle, with an effusion, which he had had for nearly 12 months. He had been losing weight and was obviously chronically unwell.

He had TB of his ankle, which, by the time he was seen, had severe, irreversible arthritic changes.

In the long run, a clear, coherent letter containing all the available and necessary information leads to a safer, more efficient experience for the patient. Practices must keep copies of letters sent to hospitals for medico-legal purposes. Handwritten letters need to be photocopied, but all too frequently such copies are illegible. There really is no substitute for typed or word-processed letters. Most computer systems come with a word-processing system, which automatically files a copy of any letter into the patient's computerised record. There is no excuse for not using such a system in the 21st century.

Other records

Practices should remember that they must keep the following records also:

- staff employment records
- personal medical reports (PMR) for insurance purposes (6 months minimum)
- maintenance records, especially for equipment like the steriliser
- financial records.

Key questions

- Does the practice recognise the importance and clinical governance issues around sound record keeping?
- Is the practice aware that clear, coherent, comprehensive letters to colleagues have a direct bearing on continuity of patient care?

Referral letter audit

Audit the contents of about 30 letters leaving the practice to assess the quality of the practice's referral letters. Consider what standard should be reached before assessing the practice's letters and record this in the column labelled 'Pre-set standard'.

G	Analyse about 30 referral letters and record the percentage of the following data included in the referral letters		Percentage included								
			< 20%	20–30%	31–40%	41–50%	51–60%	61–70%	71–80%	81–90%	> 90%
			Score 1	Score 2	Score 3	Score 4	Score 5	Score 6	Score 7	Score 8	Score 9
1 Patient identification information		Pre-set standard									
	Name										
	Address										
	Contact telephone numbers										
	Hospital number and NHS number are useful additions										
2 Clinical information		Pre-set standard									
	Provisional diagnosis										
	Reason for referral (for example diagnostic problem, or further investigations)										
	Degree of urgency										
	History and examination findings of the problem being referred										

	Pre-set standard	Percentage included								
		< 20%	20–30%	31–40%	41–50%	51–60%	61–70%	71–80%	81–90%	> 90%
		Score 1	Score 2	Score 3	Score 4	Score 5	Score 6	Score 7	Score 8	Score 9
Relevant past medical history and ongoing problems, including disability										
Results of investigations of the problem to date										
Medication or treatment already being taken for the problem (and any which might have failed to solve the problem if appropriate)										
Other medication being taken										
Drug (and other) allergies; the severity of the allergic response might be relevant										
3 Other relevant information										
Any relevant social history, for example, if the patient lives alone (information about next of kin might be very valuable information), frequently travels abroad or has language, hearing or understanding difficulties										
Total scores										

Having completed the analysis, ask the question, 'Does the practice match up to the pre-set standards?' Consider repeating the audit after a reasonable time lapse, but improve the pre-set standards.

Clinical record audit

Carry out an audit of about 200 sets of randomly selected notes (FBA requirement). Start by stating what you believe a good standard should be for each of the following criteria and record this in the column labelled 'Pre-set standard'. Then analyse the last four Lloyd George cards (or two A4 pages).

G FBA MAP	Analyse about 200 sets of records and record the percentage of the following data included in the records. (Much of this audit is particularly relevant to those using paper records)	Pre-set standard	Percentage included								
			< 20%	20–30%	31–40%	41–50%	51–60%	61–70%	71–80%	81–90%	> 90%
			Score 1	Score 2	Score 3	Score 4	Score 5	Score 6	Score 7	Score 8	Score 9
1 What percentage of the cards (or pages) are tagged in chronological order?											
2 What percentage of the cards have the following information recorded on them (all found at the top of the FP10 card):											
(a) Name?											
(b) Date of birth?											
(c) Address?											
(d) NHS number?											
3 What percentage of entries have the following recorded:											
(a) Dates?											
(b) Location or type of consultation (surgery or telephone consultation, visit, emergency)?											
(c) Legible signature of the doctor or other clinician?											
4 *Letters*: what percentage of the letters are tagged in chronological order?											

	Pre-set standard	Percentage included								
		< 20%	20–30%	31–40%	41–50%	51–60%	61–70%	71–80%	81–90%	> 90%
		Score 1	Score 2	Score 3	Score 4	Score 5	Score 6	Score 7	Score 8	Score 9
5 *Results*: what percentage of the pathology results are tagged in chronological order?										
6 *Summaries*: what percentage of the notes are summarised with up-to-date summaries?										
7 *Drug records*: what percentage of those notes of patients on long-term medication contain drug record cards?										
Total scores										

Having completed the analysis, ask the question, 'Does the practice match up to the pre-set standards?' If so, consider improving the standard and repeating the audit in six or nine months' time to see if the standard has improved. If not, consider mechanisms for improving the standard and repeating the audit to see if the practice now matches the previously pre-set standard.

For Electronic Patient Records

Consider carrying out an audit of the quality of the content of the consultation record.

G	Analyse about 200 computer entries and record the percentage of the following data included in the records	Pre-set standard	Percentage included								
			< 20%	20–30%	31–40%	41–50%	51–60%	61–70%	71–80%	81–90%	> 90%
			Score 1	Score 2	Score 3	Score 4	Score 5	Score 6	Score 7	Score 8	Score 9
1 A specific diagnosis											
(a)	Relevant history										
(b)	Relevant examination										
(c)	Treatment offered										
(d)	What the patient was told										
2 *Summaries*: what percentage have up-to-date summaries?											
			> 90%	81–90%	71–80%	61–70%	51–60%	41–50%	31–40%	20–30%	< 20%
			Score 1	Score 2	Score 3	Score 4	Score 5	Score 6	Score 7	Score 8	Score 9
3 What percentage of the summaries are cluttered with unnecessary minor diagnoses?											
Total scores											

Reference

1   General Practitioners Committee and Royal College of General Practitioners (2000) *Good Medical Practice for General Practitioners*. GPC and RCGP, London.

Record keeping and letters

Patients' records

		No	Partially	Yes, completely
ToS	Does the practice consider itself 'paperless'?	No	Partially	Yes, completely
ToS	Does the practice have written **consent from the health authority** that it fulfils the criteria as laid out in the Terms of Service for 'computerised records', paragraph 36 (amended 1 October 2000)?		No	Yes
ToS	Is the practice aware of the guidelines, '**Good Practice Guidelines for General Practice Electronic Patient Records**', prepared by The Joint Computing Group of the GPC and the RCGP (available on the Department of Health website)?		No	Yes
MAP/FBA	Has the practice ever audited the **quality of the patients'** records?	No	Yes, once within the last three years	Yes, this is regularly undergone, as the quality of record keeping is seen as an important part of: • the clinical governance agenda • continuity of patient care • protection for clinical staff in the event of a complaint or litigation
What score did the practice score in the *written* clinical records audit?		Score 1	Score 2	Score 3	Score 4	Score 5	Score 6	Score 7	Score 8	Score 9
What score did the practice score in the *computer* clinical records audit?		Score 1	Score 2	Score 3	Score 4	Score 5	Score 6	Score 7	Score 8	Score 9

L	Does the practice have a policy to allow patients **access to their records?**	No			Yes, but it is not written down and easily accessible			Yes, it is referred to in the practice leaflet, and there is a copy of the policy easily accessible to the practice staff so that should a patient ask for access to their notes, the staff can refer to it and advise the patient accordingly		
		Score 1	Score 2	Score 3	Score 4	Score 5	Score 6	Score 7	Score 8	Score 9
	Are *all* **records of out-of-hours consultations** sent to the practice within 24 hours of taking place and stored chronologically in the patients' records (or entered onto the computer records)?	No			Yes			Yes, and the standards agreed with the out-of-hours service are monitored and recorded to ensure that they are met at least 75% of the time		
		Score 1	Score 2	Score 3	Score 4	Score 5	Score 6	Score 7	Score 8	Score 9
	Do all the **clinical members** of the practice team have access to the medical records?	No			Yes, all clinical staff all of the time			Yes, but there are built-in restrictions for particularly sensitive areas by using specific security levels within the computer systems		
		Score 1	Score 2	Score 3	Score 4	Score 5	Score 6	Score 7	Score 8	Score 9

	Score 1	Score 2	Score 3	Score 4	Score 5	Score 6	Score 7	Score 8	Score 9
L E Is the practice aware of the Data Protection Act 1998?	No			Yes, but it is not referred to in the policy allowing access to the notes			Yes, the practice is aware that this applies to all records (written and computerised), and it is referred to in the policy for allowing patients access to their notes. The Access to Health Records Act 1990 is also referred to		
L E Is the practice aware of the Access to Health Records Act 1990?	No			Yes, but the practice is unaware of when it applies in light of the Data Protection Act			Yes, the practice refers to the fact that access to notes held on *deceased* patients still comes under the Access to Health Records Act 1990. As such, next of kin can only have access to the records of their deceased relative from 1 November 1991 onwards. This is highlighted in the practice policy allowing access to patients' records		

Referral letters

What score did the practice achieve in the **referral letter audit?**	Score 1	Score 2	Score 3	Score 4	Score 5	Score 6	Score 7	Score 8	Score 9
Total score, count the number of criteria scoring 1 and place the total in the first box, then the number scoring 2 and place in the second box and continue with scores 3, 4, 5, 6, 7, 8 and 9	The areas scoring 1, 2 or 3 **urgently** need to be put in place or need significant improvement			The areas scoring 4, 5 or 6 need reviewing and improving			The areas which are working well score 7, 8 or 9. Can the principles of these systems be transferred to other areas of practice work?		
Total scores	**Score 1**	**Score 2**	**Score 3**	**Score 4**	**Score 5**	**Score 6**	**Score 7**	**Score 8**	**Score 9**

L = legal requirement
G = considered good practice
MAP = Membership of the RCGP by Assessment of Performance

ToS = contractual or in Terms of Service
QTD = Quality Team Development

E = essential for revalidation
QPA = Quality Practice Award
FBA = Fellowship of the RCGP by Assessment of Performance

PART THREE
PRACTICE MANAGEMENT
POLICIES, STAFF AND EDUCATION

If a man will begin with certainties, he shall end in doubts; but if he will be content to begin with doubts, he will end in certainties.

Francis Bacon 1561–1626

9

Management policies, clinical governance and risk management

Background

By far the majority of practices in the UK are privately owned small businesses. Most are well established and have been seeing patients in much the same way for many years. A few governmental pressures have altered the emphasis on healthcare delivery; payment and incentive schemes have altered priorities. Fundamentally, however, the system of seeing patients on request, two surgeries per day with or without an appointment is the same as it has been for many years.

What has changed beyond recognition is the pressure and demands on primary care and as such, good practice management has been an essential component of the practice machinery. It is now the case that in order that a practice can work safely, effectively and efficiently, systems need to be developed and implemented. The most essential part of the implementation process is clear instructions for those who use these systems.

Why bother to develop policies within an organisation? Writing policies, I would argue, gives those developing them time to really consider all the implications of the system under development, and further, it means that those who are affected by it can refer to the written policy when necessary. It is usually at a most critical moment that referral to a policy document is necessary; for example, where does the recently recruited receptionist turn for immediate help when the duty doctor has gone out on an urgent visit, the other doctors are not available for various reasons and a patient is brought into the surgery critically ill?

There are also legal obligations on practices to produce some policies. For example, all practices employing more than five staff must have a Health and Safety at Work policy; since 1996, all practices are obliged to have a complaints procedure.

The relatives of a patient who had died of disseminated cancer complained that their father had suffered unnecessary pain during the last months of his life due to a failure of the GP to make the diagnosis soon enough.

At an independent review the doctor was asked why he had failed to respond to an abnormal blood test that had been taken at the onset of the patient's back pain. This was six months before the diagnosis was finally made. It transpired that the blood test had been filed without the doctor seeing it.

The independent review panel then started asking questions about the practice's policy for filing results. The discomfort of the doctor was very apparent when it was clear that the GP was making up the policy on the spot. The GP was even more uncomfortable when the practice receptionist was asked the same question and gave a completely different answer.

Not only was the doctor highly criticised for the absence of a clear results filing policy, but failure to deal with the complaint appropriately and the lack of a complaints policy was equally criticised.

Much legislation related to general practice is based on patient safety and protection of staff. It is not put in place just to make our jobs harder, as it sometimes seems!

Despite the fact that the drafting of policies and procedures can be tedious and time-consuming, most good practice managers will be aware that it is now an essential part of practice life. In the long run it is a valuable proactive feature of practice work and, arguably, can be nearly as important to patient care as sitting in front of the patients. In some instances it compares with using evidence-based guidelines to treat clinical conditions; for example, sound sterilisation and infection control policies protect patients from acquiring infections during invasive procedures at the surgery; and also protect the doctor from being sued. An attitude of 'It won't happen to me!' is blatant complacency.

To make the process of writing policies easier, many practice managers will have policies they have written or come across in other surgeries where they have worked. Networking with neighbouring practices can lead to a reduction in work and a cross-fertilisation of ideas. Furthermore, most health authorities and primary care organisations (PCO) have 'off-the-shelf' policies covering areas like Health and Safety at Work and Good Employment Practices, which can easily be adapted for use in the surgery. Before setting out to write any policy, enquire whether local practices or the PCO have a policy available to adapt.

There is little point in developing policies or procedures and then hiding them in the practice manager's office. Policies must be available to those who will need access to them. For example, policies relating to the work of the reception staff, like the complaints procedure, should be kept in a folder at the reception desk.

Likewise, staff must be made aware of the policies relating to the way they work, which should include any necessary training for staff. An introduction to a policy and procedure folder should be part of any staff induction programme. Some practices get staff to sign that they have read the policy folder (that is, those parts that affect them), and then insist that they update themselves every year.

The questions in this chapter cover policies not covered elsewhere in the book.

Clinical governance and risk management

All of us take risks every day. Risk management is a process which accepts that life is full of risks. It attempts to eliminate unnecessary risks and to reduce necessary risks to an acceptable level. The principles of clinical risk management mirror this. It forms one of the cornerstones of clinical governance. An assessment of clinical risk management policies forms a major part of the clinical governance review carried out by the CHI.

Without necessarily making the connection, most of us already understand the principles behind risk management. Few of us drive around with bald tyres on the car; without road tax or motor insurance; without getting the car serviced at regular intervals. Subconsciously, we assess the risk of not replacing the tyres or getting the car taxed and insured or failing to get it serviced. We make the decision that the risk of not doing these things is too great. That risk may be to our own safety, or of being caught on the wrong side of the law, or just of being stranded in the middle of nowhere.

In fact, during any single day, many subconscious issues may be considered; the risks for and against a certain decision are assessed and the final decision made, based on the lowest possible risk of something going wrong.

There are, of course, risk takers. Those who drive around with bald tyres, hoping that they are not caught and prosecuted, or that they will not have to brake hard in the rain to avoid a child. Sometimes these people, as inferred in this example, put others at risk, as well as themselves.

The nature of medicine is that it is a relatively high-risk occupation. Most of the decisions made by doctors affect others rather than themselves. Compared with general practice, some areas of medicine put patients at far greater risk, for example neurosurgery or cardiovascular surgery. All the same, in general practice we do put our patients at significant risk, for example, from the treatments we prescribe. Clinical risk management tries to minimise risks for patients. Two pillars of clinical risk management are risk assessment and incident monitoring. The third, major disaster planning, is not considered in this book.

Risk assessment

The key to reducing risks for patients is to understand those risks inherent in some systems. By carrying out an objective evaluation of the systems and treatment, or 'risk assessment', high risks can be reduced to acceptable levels and unnecessary risks removed altogether.

In general practice, one of the highest-risk procedures is prescribing. Much of the risk assessment process is done for us. Drug companies carry out extensive assessment of drugs before they are released on to the market, thereby reducing the risk to our patients. It is our job, however, to ensure that the risks of advising any treatment for a patient are assessed before handing over the prescription; we should ensure that the patient isn't known to be allergic to a drug we might wish to prescribe or to one very similar, or that he or she isn't taking a drug known to interact with the one about to be prescribed. Here we are helped by computer systems, which give warnings of patients' drug allergies and interactions with other drugs already taken by patients.

Another risk is referral to hospital. One might argue that it is a surgeon's responsibility to explain the possible risks of surgery to patients, but I wonder how many patients fully understand the risks before the anaesthetic is given.

Policies and procedures adopted by the practice should incorporate mechanisms for assessing and reducing the risks to patients and staff whenever possible. The development of sound evidence-based guidelines and protocols for dealing with clinical problems, especially medical emergencies, is a good example of risk management, where risk assessment is usually incorporated within the guideline.

An example of another policy, which might include risk assessment, would be one for minor surgical procedures. A list of the risks to be discussed with the patient might include postoperative haemorrhage, wound infection and scarring. A policy should include a method for monitoring the practice's statistics for such complications so that an informed discussion with patients can take place. If the policy includes infection control procedures and disposal of sharp implements and clinical waste procedures, then immediately the risks to staff and patients are reduced.

Incident monitoring and event reporting

The second important aspect of clinical risk management is to accept that untoward incidents will occur. If we accept this, but learn from these incidents, then systems can be adjusted to reduce risks further. This obviously entails a mechanism of reporting incidents and discussion of these by the team.

Many practices have developed 'significant event reporting' systems. All staff are encouraged to report events, both positive and negative; as much can be learnt from positive events and good practice as negative ones. However, it is the negative ones that we are now being encouraged to report to our PCO so that others can learn from them also. It is also an obligation to report serious untoward incidents.

The principle behind any event reporting system is that for every major catastrophe there are 29 near misses and 300 minor episodes, where no injury occurred, similar to the near misses. This is known as the Heinrich Ratio (after Heinrich, 1941).[1] An example of this was shown following the 1998 Paddington train disaster, when two trains collided. After the disaster, the press interviewed several train drivers who claimed to have driven through a red light at the same point because of difficulty seeing the light. At the time it was argued that had these reports been acted upon before the disaster, it is just possible that the disaster might have been averted.

Development of a serious untoward event

The GMC document *Good Medical Practice* highlights a doctor's responsibility to learn from untoward incidents. The quality initiatives of the RCGP, Quality Team Development (QTD), Quality Practice Award (QPA), Membership and Fellowship by Assessment of Performance (MAP and FBA), all require a significant event monitoring system to be in place and used, so that the whole team can learn from each others' good practice and errors.

Aim of a significant event reporting and monitoring system

The main aim of a significant event reporting and monitoring system is to **prevent a recurrence of the event**. As a starting point, all members of the team should be encouraged to report events that have affected patient care. An event should be considered if:

- it enhanced the experience or care of a patient
- something could have been done better
- a patient was failed or harmed.

These events should be discussed in a non-threatening way at regular meetings, so that the whole team learns from the experience of others. It is essential that all practice and PHCT members are involved. Practices have found that these discussions have improved relationships between team members. A policy on significant event reporting must include:

- an easily accessible recording system
- a clearly worded 'fair blame culture'; staff do need to be aware that a totally 'blame free' culture is unrealistic. Should a member of the team be blatantly negligent or seriously lacking in skills or knowledge, this has to be dealt with in the appropriate manner

- clear patient and staff confidentiality clauses. There is one proviso to this, and that is that each and every one of us working in the NHS has a legal obligation to report serious untoward events to a higher authority; for most PHCTs this authority is the PCT (or LHG in Wales). In some cases, it may be considered the General Medical Council (GMC) for doctors and the United Kingdom Central Council (UKCC) for nurses, health visitors and midwives
- an attempt to define 'significant events', 'serious untoward incidents' or 'near misses' would be appropriate, but definitions should not be too rigid, as experience of other practices and PCTs has shown that rigid definitions tend to deter people from reporting events from which others could learn. A simple definition of 'significant event' might be 'an experience that any member of staff feels others could learn from – good or bad'. An 'untoward incident' could be any incident where a patient was harmed or could have been if action hadn't been taken to avert it. Any incident that plays on someone's mind should be discussed
- regular, minuted meetings to discuss events recorded in the recording system
- a system administrator (likely to be the practice manager)
- a clearly worded paragraph setting out the aim of discussion, in order to learn from the experience and develop a system that will either promote good practice or ensure negative events don't happen again
- each event acted upon must have a person responsible for ensuring that the changes discussed are acted upon (not necessarily the practice manager, usually the person who initiated discussion)
- each event must be reappraised after a time set at the initial discussion meeting to ensure the changes agreed have been acted upon
- the meeting should consider whether the event should be publicised further afield to other PHCTs
- all 'serious untoward incidents' must be reported to the PCO.

Most practices that have adopted such a system have found the process stimulating and educational.

Other policies and procedures the practice should have in place include (some are covered in other chapters):

- complaints procedures
- infection control policies including:
  - Control of Substances Hazardous to Health (CoSHH)
- access to records and report policy (Chapter 4)
- records and notes policy (Chapter 8)
- IT policy (Chapter 12), including:
  - Electronic Patient Record policy
  - data back-up policy
  - data protection and confidentiality policy

- staff and staff management policies (Chapter 10), including:
  - Health and Safety at Work policy
  - discrimination policies
- clinical and disease management policies and guidelines (Chapter 6)
- repeat prescribing policy (Chapter 7).

Key questions

- Does the practice understand the importance of having clear policies for the management of many aspects of practice work?
- Has the practice undertaken a programme of clinical risk management and risk assessment?
- Does the practice have a commitment to learn from untoward incidents?

Reference

1 Department of Health (2000) *An Organisation with a Memory*. DoH, London.

Management policies, clinical governance and risk management

		Score 1	Score 2	Score 3	Score 4	Score 5	Score 6	Score 7	Score 8	Score 9
ToS G MAP FBA	Does the practice produce a **practice business/development plan** every year? (Paragraph 50 of Terms of Service of The National Health Services (General Medical Services) Regulations 1992)	No			Yes, most years, but is seen as a chore not a useful document			Yes, it is seen as an essential part of practice development. It incorporates staff and doctor needs as well as service developments. It is seen as a useful way to focus the mind on the coming year and beyond		
ToS	Does the practice have a written **complaints procedure?**	No. The attitude is that complaints are nothing but a nuisance and complainants are rapidly removed from the practice list			Yes, we have the one sent by the health authority in 1996. The attitude is that complaints are an unnecessary distraction from dealing with non-complaining patients			Yes. It is under constant review, and includes timescales and deadlines for reviewing the issues raised by the complaint. It feeds into the significant event monitoring policy, thereby allowing the practice to learn from complaints. The practice has had patient input into developing the policy and feels it reflects how seriously the practice views complaints		

			Score 1	Score 2	Score 3		Score 4	Score 5	Score 6		Score 7	Score 8	Score 9
ToS	Is a copy of the complaints procedure available to give **to patients**?	No				Yes, but it is out of date				Yes. It clearly explains the patients' rights and what to expect should they file a complaint. It is translated into several languages, appropriate to those spoken in the locality			
E	Does the practice have a policy about **accepting new patients** on to the practice list?	No. The receptionist assesses patients and the decision is left solely to his or her discretion				Yes. But the practice has restrictive clauses about whether patients are assessed by a doctor before acceptance, and will only be accepted if they turn up for a New Patient Medical				Yes. The policy has clear non-discrimination clauses, but does restrict acceptance on to the list to those patients living inside the defined practice area. Staff are clearly instructed about the importance of New Patient Medicals but the policy does not insist that patients turn up for their medical			
			Score 1	Score 2	Score 3		Score 4	Score 5	Score 6		Score 7	Score 8	Score 9

		Score 1	Score 2	Score 3	Score 4	Score 5	Score 6	Score 7	Score 8	Score 9
E	Does the practice have a written policy for **removal of patients** from the practice list?	No, but all patients who do not fit in with the practice procedures are removed. Rudeness and aggression are also reasons for removal from the list			Yes, it includes reasons such as rudeness and aggression, failure to turn up for appointments and making complaints			Yes. It is included as part of our practice patient information leaflet and clearly sets out those reasons the practice considers it reasonable to remove patients from the list. It shows some flexibility and is in no way aggressive or threatening. The practice policy is to write to patients explaining that if certain behaviour continues, the practice has the right to remove them from the list. The practice always writes to a patient who has been removed from the list to explain why		
G	Does the practice write a letter of explanation to the patient following removal from the list?	No			Sometimes			Always		

	Score 1	Score 2	Score 3	Score 4	Score 5	Score 6	Score 7	Score 8	Score 9
E Does the practice have a policy to **help patients with special needs** (for example, patients with physical, hearing or visual disability, or communication impairments)?	No			Yes, but it is not fully comprehensive			Yes. It is regularly reviewed and there was patient input in writing this policy. Staff are trained in the implications of the policy and are aware that the practice ethos is one of ensuring that patients are offered as much help as possible		
Is the policy advertised in the **practice leaflet** or at the surgery?	There is no policy			No			Yes. It is well advertised and the practice keeps a record of how frequently the policy is referred to		
L Does the practice actually practise an **equal opportunities policy?**	No			Yes			Yes. In fact, the practice has a diversity policy which actively encourages diversity among staff		

Comments and notes:

		Score 1	Score 2	Score 3	Score 4	Score 5	Score 6	Score 7	Score 8	Score 9
E	Does the practice have a written policy for dealing **with test results**? Ask the staff for their views as to how clear the policy is and who they would approach in the event that the clinician who ordered the test is away from the practice	No			Yes, but it was written a long time ago and has not been reviewed for a long time			Yes, it is available for the staff to refer to when necessary. It is reviewed regularly and clearly sets out the way results are handled by reception staff. It is clear who has responsibility for ensuring that all results are assessed rapidly, even when the clinician who ordered the test is not available. It clearly sets out what happens to the result once a clinician has assessed it		
	Does the practice have a written policy for handling **abnormal results**?	No, it is assumed that a doctor will handle the result			Yes. It seems to work without problems but has never been audited or checked. The staff are never asked for their opinion about its functioning. Ultimately, the doctor who ordered the test takes responsibility for the test result			Yes. The policy is very clear about whose responsibility it is to inform the patient and how the patient is informed. It also clearly sets out how the practice reacts should the patient fail to respond to the fact that they have had an abnormal result. The policy has time frames for responses and actions to be taken. It has been audited and tested. There is a fail-safe mechanism, which highlights that a patient has failed to respond to communication about an abnormal result		

Is the practice linked to the local laboratory to receive **test results electronically?**	No			Yes, but no written policy for dealing with results has been drawn up yet			Yes. This has been included in our results policy and the responsibilities for checking results have been clarified. No result comes into the practice without being seen by a clinician		
	Score 1	Score 2	Score 3	Score 4	Score 5	Score 6	Score 7	Score 8	Score 9

Comments and notes:

Health and safety policy

	Score 1	Score 2	Score 3	Score 4	Score 5	Score 6	Score 7	Score 8	Score 9
L Does the practice have a **Health and Safety policy** (a legal requirement if there are five or more employees)?	No, but we should have one	No, because there are fewer than five employees		Yes, but it is the one sent by the health authority and has not been adapted to suit the practice situation			Yes, it has been locally developed. The practice is well aware of the importance of a Health and Safety policy and do not just have one because it is a legal requirement / Despite having fewer than five employees there is still a Health and Safety policy because the practice is aware of the relevance and importance of having such a policy		
L Does the practice have a **poster** explaining the Health and Safety policy and the employee's responsibilities?	No			Yes, but it isn't very visible			Yes, it is on show in a very prominent position. New staff are shown it during their induction programme		

	Score 1	Score 2	Score 3	Score 4	Score 5	Score 6	Score 7	Score 8	Score 9
Does the Health and Safety policy have designated individual **members of staff** who have responsibility for specific tasks or working areas within the practice?	No, there is no policy			There is a policy but it does not allocate specific areas of responsibility			Yes. Each member of staff has a specific area of responsibility, which includes ensuring that other members of staff and visitors are aware of their responsibilities for Health and Safety within the practice. One senior member of the team (and a deputy in case of absence) has overall responsibility, and he or she is clearly named in the policy		
E Does the practice have a clear section in the **Health and Safety policy** (or a separate policy) referring to infection control?	No			Yes			Yes. One member of the team (the senior practice nurse) has overall responsibility for infection control, sterilisation of equipment and cleanliness of all areas, particularly those used for invasive procedures		

L		Score 1	Score 2	Score 3	Score 4	Score 5	Score 6	Score 7	Score 8	Score 9
Is there is a separate policy or a section in the Health and Safety policy referring to **Control of Substances Hazardous to Health (CoSHH) regulations?**		No			Yes, but this has not been reviewed for a long time and no one is sure who has responsibility			Yes. The responsible person is fully trained in the CoSHH regulations, and the policy includes lists of all dangerous substances kept on the premises as well as details of the correct 'post-exposure procedures' ('needle-stick' injuries)		
Are clear records kept confirming the **CoSHH** procedures are understood and followed?		No, there is no CoSHH policy			No, but there is a CoSHH policy			Yes, all records are kept up to date		
Does the CoSHH policy include who has responsibility for the disposal of **clinical waste?**		No, there is no CoSHH policy			No, but there is a CoSHH policy. Disposal of clinical waste is the responsibility of the PCO			Yes, along with a copy of the contract with the disposal company and contact details should there be a problem with collection or disposal		

		Score 1	Score 2	Score 3	Score 4	Score 5	Score 6	Score 7	Score 8	Score 9
L	Does the practice Health and Safety policy have a clear section regarding **fire safety** procedures?	No			Yes, but it is in need of being updated			Yes. One member of staff has clear responsibility to ensure that all members of staff are well versed in fire safety. Each member of staff has a responsibility to ensure that patients are assisted in the event of a fire		
L	When was the last **fire drill**?	Can't remember, or never had one			At least three years ago			Within two years. The fire brigade were involved and assisted in training staff		

		Score 1	Score 2	Score 3	Score 4	Score 5	Score 6	Score 7	Score 8	Score 9
G	How often do the staff have **fire safety training?**	Never			Occasionally and irregularly; there is no record of the last time staff underwent training			Every member of staff is given a copy of the fire safety policy when they join the practice. They also have to attend fire lectures at least once a year		
G	Are there **records** of • when the fire alarms were last tested • when a fire drill took place • which staff last attended fire safety training?	No			Yes, but they are out of date			Yes, they are clear and kept up to date		
E	Does the practice have a clear policy on staff and **practice security?**	No			Yes, but it is in need of review			Yes, all members of staff are well aware of their own as well as patient security. There are clear guidelines and training in aspects of security		

Does the practice have a **policy on violence and aggression?**	No			Yes, but it is vague and usually means that either one of the doctors, the practice manager or the police are called to deal with violent or aggressive situations			Yes. Every member of staff is well aware of their responsibility should a patient start acting in an aggressive fashion. The staff have training on how to prevent getting into a potentially confrontational situation and how to diffuse a situation that is spiralling towards aggression or violence. All staff are briefed on what to do at the first signs of violence		
	Score 1	Score 2	Score 3	Score 4	Score 5	Score 6	Score 7	Score 8	Score 9
Is there a health authority policy on prevention of **violence in primary care?**	Don't know No, definitely not			Yes, but it is of little relevance to the practice			Yes there is, and the practice policy takes this into account		
	Score 1	Score 2	Score 3	Score 4	Score 5	Score 6	Score 7	Score 8	Score 9

Risk management

E, QTD, MAP, FBA, QPA	Does the practice have a **significant event reporting** (SER) and monitoring system?	No			Yes, but rarely used			Yes, regularly used and regularly discussed and monitored		
		Score 1	Score 2	Score 3	Score 4	Score 5	Score 6	Score 7	Score 8	Score 9
	Does the SER system include **clinical events**?	There is no SER system			The SER system does not include clinical events			Yes, the system does include clinical events. The monitoring of the system feeds into clinicians' personal professional development plans to ensure that lessons are learnt and the system is backed by education		
		Score 1	Score 2	Score 3	Score 4	Score 5	Score 6	Score 7	Score 8	Score 9
	Does the SER system include **administrative events**, which, while they did not directly affect patient care, might have impacted on the staff involved and, therefore, could affect patients' care indirectly?	There is no SER system			The SER system does not include these kinds of events			Yes, all such events are recorded and acted upon. The staff involved have the opportunity to comment and, therefore, learn from the event. The aim of the SER system is to prevent a recurrence of the event		
		Score 1	Score 2	Score 3	Score 4	Score 5	Score 6	Score 7	Score 8	Score 9

		Score 1	Score 2	Score 3	Score 4	Score 5	Score 6	Score 7	Score 8	Score 9
E, QTD, MAP, FBA, QPA	Does the practice encourage **discussions** of significant events **at regular meetings** (three per year)?	There is no SER system			No, we rarely discuss events			Yes, regularly. A part of the practice meeting is dedicated to significant events. The whole PHCT is involved in these meetings		
		Score 1	Score 2	Score 3	Score 4	Score 5	Score 6	Score 7	Score 8	Score 9
G	Does the practice **monitor the outcome** of events discussed, and do they go round the 'audit cycle'?	There is no SER system			No			Yes, this is an important part of the whole system, and is a key factor in ensuring that there is no recurrence of the event		
		Score 1	Score 2	Score 3	Score 4	Score 5	Score 6	Score 7	Score 8	Score 9
Total score, count the number of criteria scoring 1 and place the total in the first box, then the number scoring 2 and place in the second box and continue with scores 3, 4, 5, 6, 7, 8 and 9		The areas scoring 1, 2 or 3 **urgently** need to be put in place or need significant improvement			The areas scoring 4, 5 or 6 need reviewing and improving			The areas which are working well score 7, 8 or 9. Can the principles of these systems be transferred to other areas of practice work?		
Total scores		Score 1	Score 2	Score 3	Score 4	Score 5	Score 6	Score 7	Score 8	Score 9

L = legal requirement
G = considered good practice
MAP = Membership of the RCGP by Assessment of Performance

ToS = contractual or in Terms of Service
QTD = Quality Team Development

E = essential for revalidation
QPA = Quality Practice Award
FBA = Fellowship of the RCGP by Assessment of Performance

10

Staff employment

Background

It seems common sense that if one treats the staff well they will be happier, less stressed, perform more efficiently, treat patients pleasantly and probably improve the practice income. They are likely to be more courteous to patients and generally make the practice a better place for patients and staff alike. As such, they are less likely to generate complaints. Campbell *et al.* found that outcomes improved also; patients had better access to services and treatment of patients with type II diabetes was improved in practices where the staff reported a 'better team climate'.[1]

Unfortunately, the author has assessed practices where staff are depressed, stressed, feel undervalued and generally dislike the work they are doing. It is often an enormous relief for staff to be able to tell someone how unhappy they are.

Good employment practice

GPs are bound, like every other employer, by employment laws. Most of the legislation relates to the Employment Rights Act 1996. However, these laws are changing very rapidly at present, partly owing to the change in government in 1997, and partly as a result of European legislation.

The CHI sees staff and staff management as one of the seven pillars of clinical governance. Part of a CHI clinical governance review includes an assessment of the attitude of NHS organisations, including GPs, towards the wellbeing and development of their staff.

Furthermore, it seems likely that as employment of staff is one of the key clinical governance issues, any assessment of the practice for revalidation of doctors will include an assessment of employment practices.

The National Primary and Care Trust (NatPaCT) website, www.natpact.nhs.uk, sets out the standards expected in the human resources policy of all NHS organisations.

The author has witnessed the extremes. One practice so values the input from the staff, and fully recognises that the cleaners and receptionists are just as vital to the safe and smooth running of the practice, that the doctors not only buy lunch for the staff on duty every day, but they also have regular team-building exercises, including trips abroad.

The opposite extreme was seen in a practice where the staff had contracts that were so out of date they were the three-month, probationary contracts that they started with five years previously. They worked in a cramped, dirty, dark reception area which posed a serious risk in the event of a fire, because it was so cluttered with papers and boxes.

During the assessment, the mention of an annual appraisal was such a strange idea that most members of the staff had to have the term 'annual appraisal' explained to them. Two staff members actually asked what the law was concerning breaks during the day, because they weren't allowed a break from the moment they arrived to the moment they left.

In a third NHS practice, a member of the reception staff was expected to arrive at 8.00am amd leave at 7.00pm, without a break all day, five days per week and then carry a bleep 24 hours a day, seven days a week to make appointments for private patients to see the GP he worked for. The salary paid to this staff member was about £10 000 per year, with no overtime payments.

There are many handbooks on good employment practice and most have advice about employment law. However, the best way of getting up-to-date information about a point of law is to phone your health authority or PCO human resources department. Some health authorities have produced their own handbooks. East London and the City Health Authority,[2] for example, produced a very comprehensive handbook for GPs, which includes model contracts and job descriptions. It includes sound advice about the recruitment process, with application and interview scoring forms, and disciplinary procedures. It also has an all-inclusive list of other agencies who will advise about employment issues.

The British Medical Association (BMA) has advisors on employment issues who are always willing to advise practices on all aspects of employment, including the difficult area of discipline and sacking staff.

The questions in this section highlight some of the most important aspects of employment law and good employment practice; they are not, however, exhaustive. They are intended to explore the practice's attitude towards employment issues and show areas that would benefit from improvement.

Recruiting staff

Advertising, interviewing and appointing staff can be complex and time-consuming. Time spent ensuring that the practice has a written policy and procedure may be an investment for the future. The recruitment process must be open, and seen to be fair and non-discriminatory. Equal opportunities legislation goes back to 1944 with the Disabled Persons (Employment) Act through to the Employment Rights Act 1996. Employers need to know about the following:

- Equal Pay Act 1970
- Rehabilitation of Offenders Act 1974
- Sex Discrimination Act 1975
- Race Relations Act 1976 and Race Relations (Amendment) Act 2000
- Disability Discrimination Act 1995
- Employment Rights Act 1996.

There are also five codes of practice approved by Parliament, which offer guidance on employment procedures. While they are not enforceable in law, they are taken into account should a practice end up in an industrial tribunal.

The employment provisions within the Disability Discrimination Act (1995) came into force on 1 December 1998. Currently, they don't apply to employers who employ fewer than 15 people, but the principles are sound and should at least be considered by all small employers like GPs. They will apply to all employers from October 2004.

- Think of the value that could be gained by patients with a disability seeing a receptionist with disabilities behind the desk.
- Think of the valued input into service provision by an employee with a disability.

Likewise, how many practices are fully aware of the implications of the Race Relations Act 1976 and the Race Relations (Amendment) Act 2000 in terms of employing staff? Practices might consider having a diversity policy *and believing in it*. It will not only give practices an advantage for being able to recruit and retain new staff, but practices are likely to find that it brings about far-reaching changes in the way the practice operates. Employers who have adopted a genuine 'diversity policy' have discovered advantages way beyond their predictions.

Retaining staff

In many parts of the country, retaining good staff is a very real problem. Many surveys have shown that when it comes to job satisfaction, most employees *do not* put pay as the most important thing on the list. To be valued, appreciated, respected and to have good terms and conditions, and personal development, frequently come higher than pay.

Certainly, in inner cities, it is not difficult for good receptionists and administrative staff to get higher-paid jobs than those offered by GPs. For this reason, good employment practice is one key element to retaining good staff. Time spent ensuring that the policies that encourage good employment practices are in place is an investment. It is worthwhile finding out what helps motivate individual members of staff, to maintain morale.

Advertising, interviewing and training are extremely time-consuming and can be very costly. Invest in your existing staff instead.

Training

The questions in the table below emphasise the importance of staff training, starting with a good induction programme through to continued personal development of staff. There are many good reasons why staff should be given opportunities to develop, not least of which is showing staff that they are valued. However, there is no reason why staff development can't dovetail in with the practice development plan so that services can be enhanced also.

This in itself highlights the importance of regular staff appraisals, which should be a two-way process of discussing the personal needs of the employee and developing the future needs of the practice.

Exit interviews

Finally, find out why a member of staff is leaving. Obviously, there are many good reasons why staff leave, but if they are leaving because something has gone wrong or you are unsure why they are leaving, then find out more. There may be a problem that you have not perceived, which can then be rectified to stop more staff leaving. You may glean useful information about policies you have in place, or more importantly, ones you perhaps should have in place.

Key questions

- Does the practice recognise that staff play a key role in health outcomes for patients?
- Does the practice genuinely value the staff?
- Is the practice committed to good employment practices?

References

1   Campbell SM, Hann M, Hacker J *et al.* (2001) Identifying predictors of high quality general practice: observational study. *BMJ.* **323**: 784–7.

2   East London and the City Health Action Zone (2001) *Good Employment Practice Handbook.*

Staff employment

L	Do *all* staff have an up-to-date **contract of employment?**	No			Yes, but it hasn't been reviewed for several years			Yes. The contract is regularly reviewed and updated in line with the changes in job description and time spent at work		
		Score 1	Score 2	Score 3	Score 4	Score 5	Score 6	Score 7	Score 8	Score 9
L	Is the contract always signed by the practice and employee **within 8 weeks** of the employee starting the job?	No			Usually			Yes, always		
		Score 1	Score 2	Score 3	Score 4	Score 5	Score 6	Score 7	Score 8	Score 9

Part 1 of the contract

L	Does the contract contain the following:	No	Yes
1	Employer's name and address (practice or doctor's)		
2	Employee's name and address		
3	Accurate job title		
4	Location of post		
5	Start date		
6	Date of commencement of *continuous employment* (this may be different from the start date if an employee is changing their job)		
7	Period of employment – fixed, temporary or probationary periods clearly specified		
8	Scale of pay (and notification as to whether the employee is entitled to *London weighting*)		
9	Frequency of payment		
10	Incremental rises (*spine points*)		
11	Hours to be worked (since November 1998 the maximum is 48 hours per week)		
12	Leave entitlement (since 1999 all employees who have worked more than 13 weeks are entitled to a minimum of 4 weeks' *paid* leave)		
13	Pension arrangements (since 1 September 1997 all practice staff are entitled to join the NHS pension scheme. Practices must offer and operate the scheme for employees)		
14	Sickness pay and arrangements (including the employee's responsibilities regarding letting the practice know they are unwell)		

L	Does the contract contain the following:	No	Yes
15	Entitlement to *time off for dependants* (staff must be allowed *reasonable* time off to deal with emergencies involving a dependant)		
16	Maternity rights and pay		
17	Notice of termination of employment on both sides		
18	Retirement (make sure there is no discrimination!)		
19	Part 2 practice-specific policies and regulations		
20	Signatures of both parties		

Count the number of ticks in the 'Yes' column	Less than 14 Score 1	14 Score 2	15 Score 3	16 Score 4	17 Score 5	18 Score 6	19 Score 7	20 Score 8	20 and more items Score 9

Part 2 Other 'practice-specific' policies

(specific questions about other practice policies are asked in Chapter 9)

Does the contract contain a clause about **patient confidentiality**?	No			Yes			Yes, and as part of the induction programme the importance of confidentiality is emphasised		
	Score 1	Score 2	Score 3	Score 4	Score 5	Score 6	Score 7	Score 8	Score 9
L Does the contract have a clear **disciplinary procedure**?	No			Yes. A copy of the disciplinary procedure is given to staff when they start working at the practice			Yes. A copy of the disciplinary procedure is given to staff when they start working at the practice and the practice manager explains the procedure fully to all new members of staff during induction		
	Score 1	Score 2	Score 3	Score 4	Score 5	Score 6	Score 7	Score 8	Score 9
Does the contract contain a **grievance procedure**?	No			Yes			Yes. We are keen that all staff are aware that any grievance is dealt with promptly and fairly		
	Score 1	Score 2	Score 3	Score 4	Score 5	Score 6	Score 7	Score 8	Score 9

	Does the contract contain mention of the practice **Health and Safety at Work policy**, in particular, emphasis on the employee's responsibility to abide by the policy?	No			Yes				Yes. Part of the induction package includes awareness and training in Health and Safety matters
		Score 1	Score 2	Score 3	Score 4	Score 5	Score 6	Score 7	Score 8	Score 9
L	Do all members of staff have **job descriptions**?	No			Yes				Yes, and this is updated annually as part of the annual appraisal process
		Score 1	Score 2	Score 3	Score 4	Score 5	Score 6	Score 7	Score 8	Score 9

Comments and notes:

Recruitment

			Score 1	Score 2	Score 3	Score 4	Score 5	Score 6	Score 7	Score 8	Score 9
G	Does the practice have a written policy for **recruitment procedures**?	No				There is a policy, but it has not been reviewed for many years			Yes. This policy is regularly reviewed in line with changes in employment law and good employment practices. The process is open, fair and takes all possible precautions to avoid discriminatory practices		
L	Does the practice have any employees with a **disability**?	No, either • the practice does have more than 15 employees and should employ people with disabilities or • they haven't considered employing people with disabilities • was unaware of the laws about employing those with disabilities				No. The practice has fewer than 15 employees, but despite this has employed people with disabilities in the past			Yes. The practice has a very strict antidiscriminatory policy, which includes those with disabilities. This is not a positively inclusive policy, but an antidiscriminatory policy which works well. Those with disabilities have brought advantages to the practice for the patients and service users, as well as the staff and practice		

E	When a new member of staff is appointed are his or her **qualifications confirmed and references checked?**	No			Usually			Yes, always		
		Score 1	Score 2	Score 3	Score 4	Score 5	Score 6	Score 7	Score 8	Score 9
L	For staff who have contact with children, especially clinical staff including locum nurses and doctors, are their names *always* checked against the **Protection of Children Act List (POCAL)?**	No			Sometimes, but we don't include locum staff			Yes, this is always carried out as a matter of policy		
		Score 1	Score 2	Score 3	Score 4	Score 5	Score 6	Score 7	Score 8	Score 9

The **Protection Of Children Act (1999)** came into force in October 2000. It has, therefore, been a legal obligation since then to check that all staff members who have direct contact with children are not on the Protection of Children Act List (POCAL). A member of the practice registered with the Home Office can do this on-line. It is a very quick procedure and local police stations can give you details of how to get registered to be able to carry out this check. Further guidance is available from Her Majesty's Stationery Offices

Retention of staff

		Score 1	Score 2	Score 3		Score 4	Score 5	Score 6		Score 7	Score 8	Score 9
	What is the **staff turnover**?	Very high. Staff rarely stay more than 12 months			Moderate. Most staff have worked for the practice more than 12 months				Low. Most members of staff stay many years and have a strong sense of loyalty towards the practice			
		Score 1	Score 2	Score 3		Score 4	Score 5	Score 6		Score 7	Score 8	Score 9
G	Is the practice aware of the value of retaining staff?	No. The staff turnover is very high and policies do not show staff that they are valued			Yes, but this isn't really borne out by some practice policies, and the staff turnover is fairly high				Yes. All staff policies are aimed at ensuring good employment practices, and staff feel valued			
		Score 1	Score 2	Score 3		Score 4	Score 5	Score 6		Score 7	Score 8	Score 9

Staff training

E	**Induction programme:** do all new staff go through an induction programme?	No, but the other staff are expected to show the new staff member 'the ropes'			Yes, but this is informal and not pre-planned			Yes. All new staff members are given a written plan of the induction programme. It explains what is covered in the induction programme, what they are expected to learn and who will teach them. It also includes clear discussion of the contract, especially the part on practice-specific policies, the Health and Safety policy and procedures; their job description and the attitude and ethos of the practice including confidentiality. It gives them ample opportunity to ask questions about issues or problems they may have		
		Score 1	Score 2	Score 3	Score 4	Score 5	Score 6	Score 7	Score 8	Score 9
	Continuing training: is **on-site training** carried out formally and a record kept?	No, it is informal and ad hoc			Formal training takes place on-site, but is not recorded or reviewed			Formal training takes place on-site. A planned programme is given to staff members at the start of employment, and reviewed at the annual appraisal. It is based on practice as well as staff needs. It is always recorded in the staff record		
		Score 1	Score 2	Score 3	Score 4	Score 5	Score 6	Score 7	Score 8	Score 9

	No, they tend to be discouraged, usually on the grounds of cost			Usually supported, but not *actively* encouraged			Yes, this is seen as an essential part of personal *and practice* development		
Are staff actively encouraged to go on **outside courses**?	Score 1	Score 2	Score 3	Score 4	Score 5	Score 6	Score 7	Score 8	Score 9
E — Are the practice nurses specifically encouraged to attend **clinical training courses**?	No			Yes, but there is no formal assessment of which courses are attended			Yes. The practice and the individual's personal developmental needs are assessed, and courses prioritised accordingly		
	Score 1	Score 2	Score 3	Score 4	Score 5	Score 6	Score 7	Score 8	Score 9
G — Do administrative staff and nurses regularly undergo **appraisals**? Do all employed staff including nurses and practice manager undergo **appraisals**?	No			Yes, but the process is not linked with the practice development plan			Yes. Staff are encouraged to discuss their own needs during the appraisal and these are linked in with the practice development plan and needs of the practice, in order that the practice can continue to offer sound comprehensive services		
	Score 1	Score 2	Score 3	Score 4	Score 5	Score 6	Score 7	Score 8	Score 9

	Low			Reasonable			High		
	Score 1	Score 2	Score 3	Score 4	Score 5	Score 6	Score 7	Score 8	Score 9
How high is **staff morale**? (Make an assessment yourself and then ask the staff to *honestly* answer this question)	Low			Reasonable			High		

Ask the staff how morale might be improved

	Score 1	Score 2	Score 3	Score 4	Score 5	Score 6	Score 7	Score 8	Score 9
G How often does the practice have **social events**, outside work?	Never or rarely			Every Christmas and perhaps once more during the year, but the same members of staff tend not to attend			Regularly, and nearly all members of staff including attached staff attend most events		
G Do staff have access to a confidential **counselling service and occupational health**?	No			Yes, but it is never or rarely used and is not well understood by staff			Yes. It is well known about by staff and has been used appropriately		

		There is no policy in place			There is a policy in place, but when staff were asked, they were not sure what they should do in the event of a 'needle-stick' injury			Yes. The policy is well documented and a poster is situated in an appropriate place with the necessary immediate action clearly advertised		
E	Do the clinical staff know what to do in the event of a **needle-stick injury**?									
		Score 1	Score 2	Score 3	Score 4	Score 5	Score 6	Score 7	Score 8	Score 9

Comments and notes:

Staff attitude

E	Do the staff nearly always maintain a **cheerful and professional attitude** towards patients? (Stand and listen to the staff during a busy Monday morning, and ask patients for their views)	Sometimes			Most of the time			Most of the time. Training sessions and staff meetings often focus on attitude towards patients and difficulties staff may have with patients at times. The issues and difficulties are openly discussed and staff offered assistance if they perceive undue difficulties. Rudeness towards patients is deemed a disciplinary matter. There are mechanisms for staff to openly discuss the fact that they felt that a doctor treated a patient rudely or discourteously		
		Score 1	Score 2	Score 3	Score 4	Score 5	Score 6	Score 7	Score 8	Score 9

		Score 1	Score 2	Score 3	Score 4	Score 5	Score 6	Score 7	Score 8	Score 9
G	Are the staff **helpful to patients** most of the time? (Consider asking the patients this question)	Yes			Yes. We have a policy of ensuring that staff see the importance of being helpful to patients			Yes. It is made clear during the induction programme that the practice ethos is one where courtesy, patient safety and satisfaction are paramount, and that we expect this to be reflected in the way staff put themselves out to help patients as much as possible. If they can't help a patient, for whatever reason, they know exactly who the patient should see in order for their problem to be resolved		
	Total score, count the number of criteria scoring 1 and place the total in the first box, then the number scoring 2 and place box in the second box and continue with scores 3, 4, 5, 6, 7, 8 and 9	The areas scoring 1, 2 or 3 **urgently** need to be put in place or need significant improvement			The areas scoring 4, 5 or 6 need reviewing and improving			The areas which are working well score 7, 8 or 9. Can the principles of these systems be transferred to other areas of practice work?		
Total scores		Score 1	Score 2	Score 3	Score 4	Score 5	Score 6	Score 7	Score 8	Score 9

L = legal requirement
G = considered good practice
MAP = Membership of the RCGP by Assessment of Performance

ToS = contractual or in Terms of Service
QTD = Quality Team Development

E = essential for revalidation
QPA = Quality Practice Award
FBA = Fellowship of the RCGP by Assessment of Performance

11

Communication and team working

It is argued that 'Communication is the most powerful tool in clinical practice'.[1] Indeed, research has shown that communication skills directly influence clinical outcomes. Furthermore, Lester and Smith demonstrated that negative communication led to an increased rate of litigation.[2] Those who work with complaints against health professionals soon learn that, within most complaints, there is an attitudinal element or a breakdown in communication between professional and patient, which forms a major component to the complaint. In fact, in terms of risk management, an assessment of communication skills of the whole team would be a true investment.

All measures of quality of health systems include an assessment of team working. Likewise, all books on clinical governance suggest ways of improving health outcomes by designing models of multidisciplinary team working, like integrated care pathways. David Hands in *Clinical Governance, Making it Happen*,[3] argues that 'integrated care' is the key to improvements in efficiency and effectiveness. He explores the concept of integration in great depth.

Without regular, efficient communication systems within any team, it can barely be considered a '*team*'. PHCTs are no different. In fact, one could argue that a disseminated community team of professionals from many clinical and non-clinical areas (like social workers) now found in the primary care setting needs to have more robust channels of communication than those found in a hospital setting, where the office of the social work team or physiotherapist is just down the corridor from the patient's bed. Compare that with the district nurse's office that is 20 miles from the surgery, which is itself five miles, on the other side of a river, from the 'service user's' home as might be the case in primary care. There is little doubt that continuity of patient care is dependent on good communication between all those involved in providing that care.

The questions in this chapter explore a few of the most important channels of communication within and outwith the practice. They should be sound and efficient in order to optimise patient care. Once again, I would argue that good patient care is dependent on the quality of management systems in place.

Background

The GMC publication *Good Medical Practice*[4] spells out the responsibility that doctors have in delegating and transferring some or all of the responsibility for a patient's care to other professionals (para. 40). It also points out that increasingly, multidisciplinary teams provide the total healthcare package (para. 30).

> You should make sure that your patients and colleagues understand your role and responsibilities in the team, your professional status and specialty.

Further, there is no doubt that primary and secondary care are becoming more and more dependent on members of many different professions to provide high standards of professional care in order to adequately serve patients' needs. It seems likely, therefore, that part of the revalidation process will involve an evaluation of communication and team work within practices.

Historically, communication between doctors and social workers has been frosty, to say the least. The NHS Plan (July 2000), however, provided the challenge for health and social services to work together to provide a 'one-stop health and social care service'. For this aim to be realised, good communication channels and a full understanding of roles within teams will be essential.

While working towards Membership and Fellowship of the RCGP by Assessment of Performance (MAP and FBA), candidates have to provide evidence of 'practice organisation and team working'. The criteria focus heavily on levels of communication between team members.

Clearly, all practices have different mechanisms for contacting team members working from bases outside the practice. Some practices rely on team members phoning or calling in to collect messages; others have sophisticated electronic communication aids. Electronic mechanisms are likely to be as effective as any and very fast. They are, of course, dependent not only upon the IT skills of those using the system, but also upon their reliability to pick such messages up. Furthermore, we have all at some time been frustrated by the failure of a computer at the crucial moment. It seems obvious that, whatever form of communication one uses, there should always be a backup mechanism. Dated responses confirm that the original message has been collected.

An Independent Review Panel heard a serious complaint.

A baby had died due to biliary atresia. While there was little that could have been done to save the baby, the complaint focused on the fact that there was little or no communication between the health visitor and the GP, each saying they had left messages in various places for the other. The main thrust of the final report was that the practice failed to provide adequate channels of communication and failed to ensure that messages left for other team members were acted upon.

Worse than this, because of the failure of communication between health visitor and doctor, neither was aware that the referral to the hospital was seriously delayed and that the parents weren't being informed about what was going on.

Communication with patients

While teamwork is dependent on communication, it is obvious that patient outcomes are influenced directly by communication also. However, not only are outcomes affected by communication, patients' experiences are also coloured by communication.

All GP registrars now have to undergo critical assessment of their consultation skills before finishing their training. Furthermore, a major part of the assessment for MAP and FBA is based on evaluation by external assessors of video-taped consultations, showing just how much emphasis is placed on consultation skills and communication with patients.

A book like this cannot evaluate consultation skills, but the author cannot overemphasise the value of objective skilled assessment of video-taped consultations. The local postgraduate dean will be able to put any doctor interested in doing this in touch with a GP tutor or trainer skilled in such an assessment.

At the outset of a patient contact with a practice, whether it is the first time the patient has walked through the door or picked up the phone to make an appointment, or whether it is one of a series of contacts on a regular basis for a routine service, the way the patient perceives that contact can make all the difference to the experience and ongoing relationship with the practice.

How many times have you walked into a shop and been ignored by staff standing talking? It can be so aggravating!

- Do the receptionists pass on similar messages to your patients?
- When did you last observe the receptionists at work on a busy Monday morning?

It is worth sitting in the waiting room and observing how the receptionists interact with patients.

- How well do they communicate with patients?
- What non-verbal messages do they pass on to the patient without even realising it?

Some people manage to smile and laugh all the time, irrespective of the pressure being brought to bear.

One receptionist I worked with for many years was just such a person. She had such an endearing way of telling patients that there wasn't an appointment for a fortnight that the patients really didn't seem too mind too much. Further, they really could 'hear' her smiling down the telephone line!

Of course, if your attitude to patients is brusque and unfriendly, it is likely that your staff will adopt a similar stance.

The vast majority of complaints received by health authorities about doctors contain an element primarily relating to attitude. Friendly, listening doctors seem to be able to get away with mistakes without complaints, if the patient feels that the doctor did his or her best. If the doctor is rude and uncaring, a minimal misdemeanour will be brought to the attention of the health authority.

Written communication

How helpful is your practice leaflet? Unfortunately, some practices still see the practice leaflet as a Terms of Service nuisance. It can, of course, be a very useful device to communicate many aspects of the way the practice functions and, therefore, cut down on time-consuming, unnecessary requests. While PMS contracts are not so prescriptive, Schedule 12 of the Terms of Service lists 20 features that should be recorded in the practice leaflet, although not all of these apply to every practice. For example, if a practice is a training practice or a dispensing practice, this also needs to be recorded, but clearly it will not be applicable to all practices (items 11 and 20).

While a glossy booklet may appear attractive, it is the quality of the content of the practice leaflet that is an indicator of a practice's willingness and desire to communicate with patients. It may be the cover that sells a paperback book, but it is the content of the practice leaflet that speaks to patients and service users.

Some practices have gone considerably further, by producing a series of useful leaflets on different aspects of the practice; some produce regular news sheets to explain practice developments and changes.

Patients whose first language is not English

Health authorities and PCTs in inner cities have worked hard at providing interpreting services. These are provided either by telephone link or by booking interpreters in advance. The issues of language difficulties are discussed in more depth in Chapter 4.

Communication with outside agencies

Referrals to hospitals must be the most frequent external communication undertaken by GPs. The letter to the local hospital is the 'frontispiece' of the practice. The contents of the letter and the presentation say a lot about the practice and the practitioners. It is also an area assessed for MAP and FBA of the RCGP qualifications. For MAP, practices have to submit evidence that referral letters contain all the necessary information. This is discussed in greater detail in Chapter 8. The reason for this is that the quality of referral letters can make the world of difference to the time patients wait to get to hospital and possibly the outcome of treatment overall.

GPs have complained for many years that hospitals are slow to communicate with them, but the quality of GP letters can often be left wanting also! Furthermore, for both continuity of patients' care and for medico-legal reasons, keeping copies of letters leaving the practice is also essential. Keeping copies of medical reports for a minimum of six months is a legal requirement.

An Independent Review Panel found a GP seriously in breach of paragraph 12 (2) (d) of the Terms of Service (Schedule 2 of the NHS (GMS) Regulations 1992) for failing to refer a patient with a heart murmur to the cardiologists for a pre-anaesthetic assessment.

The patient complained that he waited unnecessarily for the original operation because this referral never took place, despite several reminders to the doctor from the patient. The doctor claimed he had made the referral and that the referral had been lost by the hospital.

There was no record of the referral in the notes and certainly no copy of a referral letter – but then there weren't any copies of any referral letters. Further, he was also found to be in breach of paragraph 36, for failing to keep 'adequate records', as a result of not keeping copies of referral letters.

In Chapter 8 there is a suggested audit to assess the quality of the practice's referral letters.

Key questions

- Is the practice committed to friendly, useful and purposeful communication with patients, without discrimination?
- Is the practice committed to optimal multidisciplinary teamwork?
- Does the level of communication within and outwith the practice enhance genuine team working, leading to good patient care?
- Does the level of communication with outside agencies meet with patient needs?

References

1 Wilson J, Tingle J (1999) *Clinical Risk Modification, a route to clinical governance.* Butterworth Heinemann, Oxford.

2 Lester GW, Smith SG (1993) Listening and talking to patients. *West Journal of Medicine.* **158**: 268–72.

3 Lugon M, Secker-Walker J (eds) (1999) *Clinical Governance, Making it Happen.* Royal Society of Medicine, London.

4 General Medical Council (1998) *Good Medical Practice* (2e). GMC, London.

Communication and team working

E	Is the practice committed to **team working and building?** Ask this question to the attached staff, including all the allied health professionals	No			Yes, but there are difficulties with certain members of the team, which need to be faced			Yes. The team works well most of the time. There are good channels of communication, and leadership and responsibilities are clearly defined by all team members. There are regular formal and social events which help team building		
		Score 1	Score 2	Score 3	Score 4	Score 5	Score 6	Score 7	Score 8	Score 9
E	Are the **team members supportive** of each other, and willing to offer help and advice when necessary?	No			Yes, most of the time			Yes, all of the time. A significant element of team meetings is ensuring that team members are working within their limitations of knowledge, skills and capacity		
		Score 1	Score 2	Score 3	Score 4	Score 5	Score 6	Score 7	Score 8	Score 9
	Is there a system or process by which members of the team, that are having difficulties within the team, can discuss the problem in a **'blame-free' culture?**	No			Yes, but it is not widely known about; it is rarely or never used and has never really been tested			Yes. It is written as part of the aims and objectives of the practice; it is used appropriately and has been seen as an essential part of the maintenance of the team structure and working		
		Score 1	Score 2	Score 3	Score 4	Score 5	Score 6	Score 7	Score 8	Score 9

Team meetings

	Question	Score 1	Score 2	Score 3	Score 4	Score 5	Score 6	Score 7	Score 8	Score 9
E	**Doctor to doctor** (group practices) How frequently do the doctors meet to discuss **clinical issues?**	Rarely			Regularly, but informally and not all doctors attend the meetings			Regularly. It is seen as an essential part of the running of the practice to provide continuity of patient care, and is highly educational		
E	**Doctor(s) and practice manager** How frequently do the doctor(s) and practice manager meet formally to discuss **practice business?**	Rarely			Informally at least once a month, sometimes minutes of the meetings are recorded			A formal meeting is held regularly (minimum monthly), minutes are recorded and referred to when necessary		
E	**Doctor(s) and staff** How frequently does the doctor (or do the doctors) meet with the practice staff for business and training purposes? (Do not include social events)	Very rarely			Once or twice per year. These are informal and not usually structured			These are held regularly with a fairly formal structure, allowing staff open, free debate about the running of the practice. Some of the meetings have an educational element. These meetings are seen as an essential part of service development		

		Score 1	Score 2	Score 3	Score 4	Score 5	Score 6	Score 7	Score 8	Score 9
E	**Primary healthcare team** How often do the members of the PHCT come into the practice for team clinical or educational meetings?	The district nurses, midwives and health visitors come into the practice when asked, but rarely other than that			There is a regular meeting with all the PHCT members (including practice staff) at least every three months where patients are discussed, and there is an educational element to the meeting			All PHCT staff meet regularly to discuss specific patients, clinical issues and for educational purposes. The whole PHCT is involved in the compiling of the practice development plan and, as such, it is 'owned' by all of the team. This is seen as an essential part of team work and development		
E	**Practice staff and PHCT** Are the practice staff fully aware of the roles of the 'attached' PHCT members and other allied health professionals?	No			Yes, but regular team meetings with the rest of the PHCT would enhance team communication and coordination			Yes. A major part of the team meetings is focused on understanding ways to enhance relationships between the whole team and promote good communication		

Comments and notes:

Contacting team members and transfer of information
(emergency rotas and contacting the doctor in an emergency are dealt with in Chapter 4)

E	**Doctor(s) and PHCT** What is the mechanism for contacting a member of the PHCT in **an emergency?**	A telephone message is left if a member of the team cannot be contacted directly			There are backup mechanisms to leaving telephone messages, like a message book left with a member of practice staff. Those PHCT members not housed in the practice are expected to contact the practice to collect messages on a regular basis			The PHCT contact the practice to collect messages on a regular basis. A member of staff is charged with the responsibility of ensuring that the messages are passed on (or collected) and the response recorded. There is a policy, signed and owned by all the relevant PHCT members, regarding this, and it is shown to any new members of the team during the induction programme		
		Score 1	Score 2	Score 3	Score 4	Score 5	Score 6	Score 7	Score 8	Score 9
	What is the mechanism for contacting the PHCT with **non-urgent messages?**	Message left with receptionist			Formal book with written message signed and dated			Formal book with written message signed and dated but with a policy that all messages are signed when collected and a formal response or answer is also recorded, which is *signed and dated*		
		Score 1	Score 2	Score 3	Score 4	Score 5	Score 6	Score 7	Score 8	Score 9

E	How does the transfer of patient information to other members of the PHCT, particularly about contacts that have occurred as **emergencies or out of hours,** take place?	It is simply recorded in the patient's records for the next clinician to find when necessary		There is a specified system or book where messages are left for the appropriate doctor to pick up when next available			There is a specified system or message book, but a member of staff is charged with the responsibility of ensuring the message is received and acted upon. If not, the message is passed back to the team member initially involved so that personal communication can take place. All team members are clear about their responsibility for passing on information. The system ensures continuity of care and is audited from time to time		
		Score 1	Score 2	Score 3	Score 4	Score 5	Score 6	Score 7	Score 8	Score 9

Team communication assessment

		Score 1	Score 2	Score 3	Score 4	Score 5	Score 6	Score 7	Score 8	Score 9
G	Carry out an informal audit to assess how well the staff and PHCT are informed about communication policies. Ask the questions: • 'Are all members of the staff and PHCT aware of how to contact a specific team member?' • 'How do you know whether that team member has responded to your message?'	Very few could answer the questions adequately			Most of the staff and team members answered the questions adequately. There is room for improvement			Everyone answered the questions without difficulty and felt the systems were watertight		

Communication with patients

ToS	Does the practice leaflet contain (or do the practice leaflets cover): (16 essential Terms of Service criteria (Schedule 12))	Place a tick in the box if present
	1 Full name of all doctors	
	2 Gender of doctors	
	3 Registered medical qualifications	
	4 Date and place of first registration	
	5 Approved times of availability for all doctors	
	6 Appointments system operated	
	7 Methods of obtaining urgent and non-urgent appointments	
	8 Method of obtaining a visit	
	9 Arrangements when doctor not personally available	
	10 Method by which patients obtain a repeat prescription	
	11 Numbers of other staff and description of their roles in practice	
	12 Whether *or not* child health surveillance, contraceptive, maternity and minor surgery services are available at the surgery	
	13 Number of partners (or single-handed or job-share) and full-time or part-time commitment	
	14 Method of receiving patients' 'comments' about services	
	15 The geographical boundary of the practice area (by sketch or plan)	
	16 Whether premises have suitable facilities and access for all disabled patients	

ToS	**Specific pieces of information to be provided by some practices:**
	1 If a dispensing practice, the arrangements for dispensing
	2 If the doctor provides clinics, the frequency, duration and purpose must be included
	3 If an assistant is employed, the details of the assistant must be included (same as for all doctors, 1 to 5 above)
	4 Teaching and training practices must advertise this fact

How well does the practice patient leaflet (or do the information leaflets) fulfil the criteria?

Score 1	Score 2	Score 3	Score 4	Score 5	Score 6	Score 7	Score 8	Score 9
No leaflet	<3 items	3–6 items	7–9 items	10–12 items	13–15 items	16 or more	All criteria and more	All criteria and much more

ToS — Is the practice **telephone number** exactly correct?

Score 1	Score 2	Score 3	Score 4	Score 5	Score 6	Score 7	Score 8	Score 9
	No, it hasn't been updated since the national numbers were changed		Yes, but new numbers available for specific reasons have not been incorporated			Yes. All numbers available to patients are included. Brief details about the telephone system are included; for example, the fact that callers will be asked to press certain numbers on their phone to specify what their request might be regarding		

Does the leaflet contain **other useful information?**

Score 1	Score 2	Score 3	Score 4	Score 5	Score 6	Score 7	Score 8	Score 9
No			Yes, but very little. Patients were not asked what information they would like included			Yes. It has been extensively researched with input from patients to ensure that other information which patients find useful is included		

		Score 1	Score 2	Score 3	Score 4	Score 5	Score 6	Score 7	Score 8	Score 9
G	Is the practice leaflet available in **different languages**?	No			Yes, but not enough			Yes. Nearly all the local languages necessary		
G	Is the practice leaflet available in large print for those with **visual impairment**?	No			Yes			Yes, and it is available in Braille. It can also be made available on cassette tape		
	Has the practice asked **patients for their views** on the leaflet?	No			Yes, but the comments were not acted upon, or the leaflet hasn't been updated since then			Yes. The ideas and information were incorporated in the leaflet and made it considerably more useful		

Try asking a patient or service user for their view of the practice leaflet.

Ask:

- Does it really give you the information you need?
- How can it be improved?

	Score 1	Score 2	Score 3	Score 4	Score 5	Score 6	Score 7	Score 8	Score 9
Now score the practice on the patients' and service users' responses	Score 1	Score 2	Score 3	Score 4	Score 5	Score 6	Score 7	Score 8	Score 9

Other means of communication with patients and service users

QTD	Does the practice have **other information leaflets** available about other practice services or policies?	No or yes, but they are out of date and generally unhelpful			Yes, but some are out of date (and are mainly in English in areas with significant numbers of patients from minority ethnic communities). Generally they are helpful, but there is room for improvement. Putting one clinical team member in charge of ensuring they are kept up to date and relevant to national and local health priorities could achieve this			Yes. They are also in different languages. They are kept relevant to national and local health priorities by a member of the clinical team. Special care is taken to ensure that sensitive leaflets like information on sexually transmitted diseases or teenage pregnancy are kept in a position where they can be collected without patients in the waiting room seeing. The practice also has a regular news sheet to inform patients of practice developments. Patients are frequently asked for their views about these mechanisms of communication		
		Score 1	Score 2	Score 3	Score 4	Score 5	Score 6	Score 7	Score 8	Score 9

QTD	Are there **posters on health education** in the waiting room?	No			Yes, but they are generally out of date, of little help and only in English			Yes. There is a policy for ensuring that they are useful, up to date and focused on local and national health priorities. They are in various languages. The practice tries to focus on a specific health issue each month and change the posters accordingly		
		Score 1	Score 2	Score 3	Score 4	Score 5	Score 6	Score 7	Score 8	Score 9
QTD	Does the practice have a ready source of literature about **self-help groups** or other local agencies?	No			A few			Yes, plenty. We have a dedicated member of staff who regularly updates the file. It is easily available for patients to consult and its locations is advertised in the surgery. Furthermore, we have a computer in the surgery connected to the Internet in order for patients to access health information, especially related to self-help groups		
		Score 1	Score 2	Score 3	Score 4	Score 5	Score 6	Score 7	Score 8	Score 9

	Score 1	Score 2	Score 3	Score 4	Score 5	Score 6	Score 7	Score 8	Score 9
E **Accessing results and reports** Does the practice have a policy for communicating results of tests and investigations?	Yes, but it is not written down anywhere. Patients are expected to phone for all results			Yes. There is a written policy, but it is not advertised or easily available to the practice staff			Yes. There is a written policy, and the relevant details are given in a leaflet for patients. Despite this, cervical smear results and some other results are sent directly to the patient with an explanation on how to proceed or discuss the result with a member of the PHCT. With those results not sent to the patient, if a result hasn't been collected after a set time period the patient is automatically contacted – even if the result is normal. There is a fail-safe mechanism for ensuring that abnormal results are responded to and this includes sending letters by recorded delivery if necessary or even a visit by one of the PHCT. The practice fully understands its responsibilities		

		Score 1	Score 2	Score 3	Score 4	Score 5	Score 6	Score 7	Score 8	Score 9
E	**Staff attitude** Does part of staff training concentrate on manner and attitude of towards patients?	No			Yes, but this is not a high priority			Yes. Very high importance is placed on staff attitude and courtesy. The practice is aware that the reception staff project an important image for the practice and can make an enormous difference to patient experience. The practice believes that if patients are treated with respect and courtesy, the consultation with the doctor is more productive and the outcome better		
G	Has the practice asked **patients for their views** about communication at all levels?	No			Yes, but no changes were made as a result of the feedback			Yes. This has altered aspects of communication and levels of staff awareness of the importance of good communication		

Referral letters

(Chapter 8 has a suggested audit to carry out to assess the quality of the content of referral letters)

		Score 1	Score 2	Score 3	Score 4	Score 5	Score 6	Score 7	Score 8	Score 9
E	Are **copies** of referral letters filed in the patients' notes?	No			The majority are, but emergency or handwritten letters for acute admissions tend to get forgotten			Yes all, including emergency letters for acute admissions. All letters are tagged and chronologically filed. Alternatively, all letters are filed in the patients' computer records		
G	Are letters **typed** on headed paper?	No			Yes, the majority. Emergency letters may not be typed but a copy is filed			Yes, the vast majority are. Most doctors even use the computer to generate emergency letters, which automatically incorporate a lot of patient details and are then automatically filed in the patients' computerised records		

Comments and notes:

Total score, count the number of criteria scoring 1 and place the total in the first box, then the number scoring 2 and place in the second box and continue with scores 3, 4, 5, 6, 7, 8 and 9	The areas scoring 1, 2 or 3 **urgently** need to be put in place or need significant improvement			The areas scoring 4, 5 or 6 need reviewing and improving			The areas which are working well score 7, 8 or 9. Can the principles of these systems be transferred to other areas of practice work?		
Total scores	Score 1	Score 2	Score 3	Score 4	Score 5	Score 6	Score 7	Score 8	Score 9

L = legal requirement
G = considered good practice
MAP = Membership of the RCGP by Assessment of Performance

ToS = contractual or in Terms of Service
QTD = Quality Team Development

E = essential for revalidation
QPA = Quality Practice Award
FBA = Fellowship of the RCGP by Assessment of Performance

12

IT and computerised systems

Background

The past 20 years have seen rapid advances in the use of information technology. While general practice has been relatively slow in keeping up, most practices do now use a computer for certain functions within the practice. It is still true to say, however, that some practices significantly underutilise the system they have; a few still do not possess a clinical computer system at all.

Only in the past eight or ten years have we seen clinical IT systems which are of any real benefit to general practice, although some office systems used for keeping registration data and carrying out repetitive functions like repeat prescribing have been around a little longer.

An enormous amount of work in practices went into putting initial data on to the computer. For example, the repeat prescribing information took several months to ensure it was comprehensive and accurate. All the same, it proved to be an investment for the future.

Now there are many primary care software systems, EMIS, VAMP, Torex, Microdoc to name just a few. These are all sophisticated data storage and retrieval systems. They are designed to be user-friendly, to allow storage of patient registration and clinical information, and to provide instant access to such information during consultations or other patient interactions. Some systems have been designed by doctors, ensuring that the way the initial screens appear looks familiar to those sitting in front of the patients.

Most systems have word-processing packages attached to them in one way or another, in order that letters about patients can be typed and stored with the patient's clinical information. Computers are also ideal for running recall systems.

Most practices with computer systems are linked to their health authorities for transfer of patient registration data and passage of information for payment purposes. Some practices are also linked to their local hospitals for the purpose of receiving results from pathology departments as well as the passage of clinical information to hospital departments, thus reducing the time taken for clinical information to be passed between professionals. By being connected to the Internet, practices are linked to the vast resources of the most up-to-date medical research information available.

The NHS Plan published in January 2001, promised 'substantial investment' in IT. Targets have been set. These include a target that by 2002, NHSnet should be accessible to 100% of practices. 'By 2005, GPs and practice staff should have straightforward systems to book hospital appointments in the surgery.'

'Paperless' practices

Some practices aspire to becoming 'paperless'. By this, they mean that they record all consultations on the computer; they do not keep paper copies of letters to colleagues and they scan letters from hospitals and other sources into the computer to be added to the patient's notes.

Some practices continue to record patient consultation information both in the paper records and on the computer. In the author's opinion, this is the worst of both worlds, as neither is a complete record of the event and, even when put together, the record tends to be inadequate.

Some practices destroy letters they have scanned into the computer system. Others, wisely in my opinion, continue to store letters to the practice and investigation results in the patient's paper record. Some practices have failed to realise that, in most software systems, a scanned document is filed in such a way that the main diagnosis still has to be recorded, by hand, in the summary section of the patient's computerised record. Unless this is carried out the chronic disease register is inaccurate.

> The author assessed a practice where, for two years, all communications from outside agencies were scanned and then destroyed immediately. Unfortunately, the scanning was unreliable, especially if the letter was not put in the scanner exactly straight. The result was that many of the scanned letters were simply unreadable. It didn't seem to occur to the person responsible for scanning the document to check the result of the scanning before destroying the original!

For these reasons, the target for practices to become paperless has not proved easy to reach.

There are, furthermore, government regulations and guidelines about practices becoming 'paperless'. The amendment of the 1992 Regulations (2000 No. 2383) states that practices must obtain 'written consent' from the health authority before relying on Electronic Patient Records. To obtain this permission, practices must fulfil certain criteria:

* The computer system must be one that has been accredited by the Secretary of State according to the 'General Medical Practice Computer Systems – Requirement for Accreditation Act – RFA99'.

- The security measures, according to this act, must be enabled.
- The doctor is aware of the *Good Practice Guidelines for General Practice Electronic Patient Records*.[1]

These guidelines are invaluable, and all practices considering going down the 'paperless' route should consult these first. They are available, along with the statutory instruments, on the Department of Health website, www.doh.gov.uk, and can easily be found by searching for 'Electronic Patient Records'.

Further comprehensive guidance is available from the General Practitioners Committee of the BMA published in July 2001.[2] It is also available on the BMA website.

Computerised records

Computerised records have many advantages. Of course, they are not only legible but are always dated, one assumes, accurately; during his trial, Harold Shipman claimed to be able to deceive the audit trail on his computer system by changing the internal date of the computer.[3]

Automatically, when using a computer to record consultations, the name of the doctor is clearly recorded at the beginning of each consultation (assuming doctors do not share passwords), as is the location where the consultation is taking place (for example, in the surgery). These details are essential evidence in the event of a complaint. However, it is easy for a clinician to record in a patient's computerised records in the 'default' location, when in fact the doctor was interrupted in the middle of the surgery by a telephone call from the patient. The doctor is now recording this consultation as a 'surgery attendance' (the default location) instead of a 'telephone consultation', unless the 'type' of consultation is actively changed. Thus, the record of where the consultation took place is now inaccurate.

Many doctors do not have computer and keyboard skills, and thus feel that the computer slows them down during consultations. This may result in vital information not being recorded due to a perceived lack of time. Further, the computer is a 'sponge' for information. If this is not accurately recorded in a standardised format by all those in the practice using the computer, then it is difficult to get accurate, useful data back out.

Clinical governance

There are many clinical governance issues that should be considered when assessing the computerised systems within a practice. The questions in this chapter assess how well practices recognise and deal with some of these issues. IT systems are one of the cornerstones of the clinical governance agenda.

Audit and evaluation of clinical outcomes

Audit and monitoring of care underpin the whole notion of clinical governance. This cannot realistically be carried out without the aid of a computer. Examples of easily collected data in primary care, suitable for audit purposes, include records of appointment systems, ongoing recording of the monitoring of chronic disease management, prescribing habits and clinical outcomes.

Clinical risk management

Computers have long been used to carry out the repetitive processes undergone daily in a doctor's surgery accurately, thereby reducing mistakes. One of the first functions performed by computers in surgeries was the production of repeat prescriptions. Now, by far the majority of practices rely very heavily on their computer system for production of repeat prescriptions.

Computer-based prescribing has other advantages, including assisting in the decision-making process. By rank listing drugs from locally based formularies, computer-prescribing tools have been shown to improve drug suitability and dose accuracy.[4] Furthermore, by highlighting drug allergies and identifying potential drug interactions, computer prescribing has reduced drug errors.

Evidenced-based practice

Most computer systems have 'templates' and evidence-based guidelines to use during consultations. These can be useful prompts to remind clinicians of the latest views on treatments available, and also to remind doctors to record certain measurements for monitoring chronic illness and the use of long-term medicines. Furthermore, provided that the storage of disease-monitoring patient data is recorded in a standardised form, it can be easily accessible for audit purposes.

Potential problems

The list of clinical governance issues posed by IT systems starts with the security of the system. The physical security of the main server must be considered by practices. If the main computer system is linked to the Internet, the health authority or to the software company by a telephone line, then there is the potential for computer 'hackers' to get in.

The Data Protection Act 1998 states:

> Appropriate technical and organisational measures shall be taken against unauthorised or unlawful processing of personal data and against accidental loss or destruction of, or damage to personal data.

It is the practice's responsibility to ensure security of the system. Most software companies and medical indemnity companies are willing to advise practices about computer hardware and data security.

Furthermore, how secure is the system within the practice? How certain are the doctors and manager that the details of the clinical records are available to some staff but not others? One might argue that we are now more concerned about security and access to information on computer systems than ever we were about access to the Lloyd George handwritten notes. We also have to be very aware of the potential for abuse of the system by staff. On the one hand, allowing maximum access by clinical staff to patient records is essential for continuity of care, but on the other hand it can mean that clerical staff have easy access to highly confidential information, at the touch of a button. It is, therefore, essential that the computer system allows for different levels of access by staff.

In one very progressive practice the author assessed, a doctor, on return from his holiday, was completely dismayed to find that, according to the computer, during his absence a whole series of prescriptions had been issued and pathology results actioned under his name.

The fact that the practice manager knew the doctor's password for the computer system made this a very complicated and unpleasant issue to resolve.

Data accuracy

Next on the clinical governance list is the accuracy of the information stored. In IT circles they say, 'If you put garbage in, you get garbage out!' That couldn't be truer of clinical systems. If audit is to be carried out and the results are to be at all useful, then the accuracy of the information put into the system is paramount. Furthermore, information needs to be in a standardised format throughout the practice, if not the whole PCO, to be truly comparable.

Many practices have tried, with considerable difficulty, to ensure that all doctors stick to using standardised Read coding for recording diagnoses in order that audit can be carried out successfully. How PCOs will obtain useful data in the future with up to 150 doctors putting different Read codes into different computer systems, remains to be seen.

Data backup

The more dependent practices become on software systems, the more important it is that they have full backup procedures. Most practices back up on a daily basis. To add to the safety of this system, they make several backups and store these in different locations on the basis that it is unlikely that the whole lot would be destroyed at once if diffusely spread around town.

Staff training

Staff training at all levels is essential. It appears that the degree of staff training in computer skills is proportional to the importance placed on the use of the computer for recall, audit and other primary care functions. And this goes for the training of the doctors as well.

The questions in this section relate to the clinical governance issues surrounding the IT system in the practice.

Key questions

- Is the practice committed to using IT systems to enhance patient care?
- Is the practice fully aware of clinical governance issues in relation to the use of IT?

References

1 The Joint Computing Group of the General Practitioners' Committee and the Royal College of General Practitioners (2000) *Good Practice Guidelines for General Practice Electronic Patient Records*. www.doh.gov.uk

2 General Practitioners Committee (2001) *A Proposed Generic Scheme for Approving Paperless Practice, Guidance for GPs*. BMA, London.

3 Department of Health (2000) *Harold Shipman's Clinical Practice 1974–1998*. A clinical audit commissioned by the Chief Medical Officer. DoH, London.

4 Wyatt J, Walton R (1995) Computer based prescribing. *BMJ*. **311**: 1181–2.

IT and computerised systems

	Score 1	Score 2	Score 3	Score 4	Score 5	Score 6	Score 7	Score 8	Score 9
Which clinical software system does the practice use?									
How long has the practice had a computer system?									
Is it one of the government-approved systems?	No, or don't know								Yes
When was the software last upgraded?	Don't know			Between two and three years ago			Within the last two years. The software company regularly reviews the system and sends regular updates. The practice is informed when these updates have been sent		
Government target — Is the practice linked to **NHSnet?**	No			Yes, but it is rarely used			Yes. It is used regularly for research and educational purposes as well as communication with colleagues		
Does the practice have full access to the **Internet?**	No			Yes, but it is rarely used			Yes. It is regularly used and accessible to all staff, especially clinical staff		

Confidentiality and security

		Score 1	Score 2	Score 3	Score 4	Score 5	Score 6	Score 7	Score 8	Score 9
E	Does the practice have **different levels of security** pass for each member of staff?	No			Yes, but the staff are not encouraged to change their password frequently, and the manager (doctor) does not know whether staff exchange passwords			Yes, and these are regularly reviewed and staff are expected to regularly change their password. They are made fully aware of the importance of not sharing passwords during their induction; the staff contract highlights that deliberately sharing passwords would be deemed a serious disciplinary matter		
E	Are staff aware that they should **sign off** the computer when they are no longer using it?	No, or don't know			Yes, but this is not discussed again after induction			Yes. This is strictly adhered to; they are reminded of the importance of doing so during practice meetings		

		Score 1	Score 2	Score 3	Score 4	Score 5	Score 6	Score 7	Score 8	Score 9
E	Are staff aware of the importance of maintaining **strict computer security**?	No, or don't know			Yes, but is not in the job contract			Yes. It is a clear part of the job contract with staff. Abusing security would be deemed a serious disciplinary matter. Discussion about computer security forms an important aspect on the staff induction programme		

Comments and notes:

		Score 1	Score 2	Score 3	Score 4	Score 5	Score 6	Score 7	Score 8	Score 9
G	Is the computer **physically secured** in such a way that theft would be very difficult?	No, it is simply kept under the reception desk			Yes. It is locked in one of the offices away from the areas accessed by patients			Yes. It is physically locked to the floor and the office is locked whenever it is not in use		
G	Does the practice regularly run a **virus detector** and have appropriate anti-virus protection?	No, or don't know			Yes, but the practice has never tried the system out			Yes. The practice has had experience of virus invasion, which was detected and isolated by the anti-virus programme		

Computer backup

		Score 1	Score 2	Score 3	Score 4	Score 5	Score 6	Score 7	Score 8	Score 9
E	Does the practice regularly make **backup** copies of the data held on the computer?	No, or less than once per week			Yes, daily and several backup copies are kept in different locations			Yes. Daily backups are carried out and copies are kept off-site in several locations. The practice has had a trial computer failure and reloaded all the data from the backup disks		
E	Where are the **backup discs held**?	Never backed up, and so not necessary			On-site in the surgery			Both on-site and off-site		
G	Has the practice tried to **restart the computer with the backup discs** or carried out a procedure to mimic a complete failure of the computer with loss of patient data?	No			Yes, but the difficulties created meant that the practice will not try it again			Yes, lessons were learnt from the exercise. A policy was written with a clear procedure and has since been retried with full success. The practice is confident that minimal patient-related data would be lost in the event of total computer failure		

L	Data Protection Act								
	Is the practice registered under the **Data Protection** Act?	No, or don't know			Yes. This was carried out for us when the practice first bought our computer system			Yes. The practice has been registered since first acquiring the computer and it has been checked and reviewed within the last year	
		Score 1	Score 2	Score 3	Score 4	Score 5	Score 6	Score 7	Score 8	Score 9

Appointment system

QTD		No			Yes			Yes, and it is regularly used to: • audit the wait for routine appointments • audit the length of time spent by patients in the waiting room before their appointment
Does the practice use a computerised appointment system?								
	Score 1	Score 2	Score 3	Score 4	Score 5	Score 6	Score 7	Score 8	Score 9
G		No			Yes, sometimes			Yes, every day	
Are **paper records** of the day's appointments made in case of a computer failure?								
	Score 1	Score 2	Score 3	Score 4	Score 5	Score 6	Score 7	Score 8	Score 9

Comments and notes:

Clinical records

Code	Question	Score 1	Score 2	Score 3	Score 4	Score 5	Score 6	Score 7	Score 8	Score 9
	Is the computer used to record **consultations**? (Practices using paper records only should ignore this question)	Yes, but the practice uses a combination of both paper and computerised records			Yes, most of the time, but attached staff do not use the computer and many consultations like telephone conversations are not recorded on the computer			Yes. All clinical staff are encouraged to record consultations with patients. This is seen as an important aspect of continuity of patient care. The practice is especially careful to ensure that ad hoc conversations with patients are recorded for future reference		
QTD	Are the patients' past and ongoing medical problems recorded on the **summary screen**?	No			Yes, but not up to date			Yes. The practice makes every effort to ensure that the summary screen is kept up to date		
G	When was the accuracy of the **summary screen last audited**?	Never			Many years ago, and it was less than 60% accurate			Within the last two years, and it was at least 85% accurate		

Repeat prescribing

E	Does the practice use the **computer to generate repeat prescriptions?**	No			Yes, most of the time			Yes, all of the time. The computer is used to audit the repeat prescribing habits		
		Score 1	Score 2	Score 3	Score 4	Score 5	Score 6	Score 7	Score 8	Score 9
NSF for Older People	Does the practice use the repeat prescription system to **recall patients for medication reviews?**	No: • the practice doesn't use a computer for repeat prescribing			Yes, the computerised repeat prescribing system is used, but: • the recall facility for medication reviews is not used, or • the facility is used but not strictly adhered to			Yes, it is strictly adhered to. Repeat prescriptions are severely restricted to patients who do not comply with the medication review system. There is a strict policy about this that is advertised to patients and service users in the surgery and the practice leaflet		
		Score 1	Score 2	Score 3	Score 4	Score 5	Score 6	Score 7	Score 8	Score 9
	When was the **'medication review'** system last audited?	Never			Two years ago, or more			Within the last two years. The importance of regular medication review is clearly understood and therefore this audit is carried out regularly		
		Score 1	Score 2	Score 3	Score 4	Score 5	Score 6	Score 7	Score 8	Score 9

Comments and notes:

Acute prescribing

G	Does the practice use the computer for *all* **acute prescribing**?	No			Mostly, but prescribing carried out on home visits or handwritten prescriptions tend not to get recorded			Yes. All acute prescribing is recorded, and special effort to record handwritten prescriptions is also made		
		Score 1	Score 2	Score 3	Score 4	Score 5	Score 6	Score 7	Score 8	Score 9
QTD MBA FBA QPA	Does the practice have and use a computer-based, practice **drug formulary**?	No			Yes, but how well it is adhered to is not monitored			Yes, and its use is audited regularly, ensuring that at least 85% of prescriptions are from the formulary		
		Score 1	Score 2	Score 3	Score 4	Score 5	Score 6	Score 7	Score 8	Score 9

Chronic disease register

		Score 1	Score 2	Score 3	Score 4	Score 5	Score 6	Score 7	Score 8	Score 9
E QTD	Does the practice have a computerised **chronic disease register**?	No, the practice does not have a chronic disease register at all			Yes, but it is only about 60% accurate and Read codes need to be reviewed and standardised by those recording chronic diseases and summarising notes on to the computer			Yes. The practice has a strict policy of maintaining and updating the patient computerised summaries and, as such, the chronic disease registers are at least 85% accurate. All clinical staff are actively encouraged to keep the data up to date		
QTD MBA FBA QPA	Does the practice use the computer to enhance and **monitor the care of patients with chronic diseases**?	No: • the practice doesn't have a chronic disease register, or • the one it has is not up to date			Yes, but not on a regular basis. At present this is rather ad hoc and doesn't form part of the chronic disease management within the practice. There are no or few evidence-based chronic disease protocols in the practice, or on the computer			Yes. This is seen as an essential tool for monitoring the care offered to patients with chronic diseases. There is a dedicated member of staff ensuring that the chronic disease register is kept up to date. The evidence-based chronic disease protocols are easily accessible on the computer system in each clinical room. There is a programme of ongoing development of these		

Clinical audit

(Chapter 6 covers clinical audit in more detail)

QTD MAP FBA QPA	Does the practice use the computer to **monitor the care provided** to patients?	No			Yes, but this is rather ad hoc and there is no structured programme of audit or monitoring set up			Yes. The practice has a regular programme of audit and monitoring. This feeds into the practice development plan. All members of clinical staff are encouraged to participate and have a say in which areas are audited	
		Score 1	Score 2	Score 3	Score 4	Score 5	Score 6	Score 7	Score 8	Score 9

Comments and notes:

Item of Service links

	No			Yes			Yes, the system is regularly monitored. It is also possible to send patients' clinical information directly to other doctors when this facility is available at the recipient surgery		
Is the practice linked to the health authority or PCT for the purpose of **Item of Service claims and transfer of registration data?**									
	Score 1	Score 2	Score 3	Score 4	Score 5	Score 6	Score 7	Score 8	Score 9

Comments and notes:

Hospital links

Is the practice linked to the local hospital for the receipt of **pathology results?**	No			Yes			Yes, the system is regularly monitored. Furthermore, the practice has access to hospital departments and can refer patients using electronic means. Likewise, hospital departments can send clinical information directly to the practice. Security of the system is also regularly checked and upgraded		
	Score 1	Score 2	Score 3	Score 4	Score 5	Score 6	Score 7	Score 8	Score 9
Total score, count the number of criteria scoring 1 and place the total in the first box, then the number scoring 2 and place in the second box and continue with scores 3, 4, 5, 6, 7, 8 and 9	The areas scoring 1, 2 or 3 **urgently** need to be put in place or need significant improvement			The areas scoring 4, 5 or 6 need reviewing and improving			The areas which are working well score 7, 8 or 9. Can the principles of these systems be transferred to other areas of practice work?		
Total scores	Score 1	Score 2	Score 3	Score 4	Score 5	Score 6	Score 7	Score 8	Score 9

L = legal requirement
G = considered good practice
MAP = Membership of the RCGP by Assessment of Performance

ToS = contractual or in Terms of Service
QTD = Quality Team Development

E = essential for revalidation
QPA = Quality Practice Award
FBA = Fellowship of the RCGP by Assessment of Performance

13

Continuing medical education and personal professional development

Background

It is without question that all health professionals need to maintain their medical knowledge if they are to offer the most relevant up-to-date advice to patients. The GMC's publication *Good Medical Practice* and the GPC and RCGP document *Good Medical Practice for GPs* both emphasise this.

However, as changes in medicine take quantum leaps, it becomes almost impossible to keep completely up to date. GPs must, therefore, prioritise educational needs and spend the appropriate amount of time on them. The question then is 'how to prioritise?' How much time should GPs dedicate to keeping up to date?

In 1992, the government acknowledged that GPs needed to spend time maintaining their medical knowledge and agreed to pay the princely sum of £2000 per annum to those doctors who spent five days per year attending accredited courses. Some still argue that the government of the day reduced GPs' income by £2000 per annum and gave them another hurdle to jump to get this sum back! All the same, it was a small recognition that medical education never stops.

Subsequently, the government's 1998 White Paper *The NHS: a first class service* highlighted the fact that lifelong learning is vital to the establishment of a modern health service of the highest quality. This was followed by two more papers, *Making a Difference* and *Supporting Doctors, Protecting Patients*, which confirmed the government's agenda, supporting continuing education for all health professionals. These papers also reiterate that doctors are going to have to go through a process of reaccreditation in order to continue to practice.

Revalidation and clinical governance

Revalidation of GMC registration for GPs is going to take into account many of the practice's management systems, as described throughout this book. Of course, proof of continuing medical education will also form a significant part. The overall process will be in three stages.

- First, doctors will have to collect information about the work they do and their performance in a 'folder'. Appraisal forms to complete are now posted on the DoH website.
- Second, this folder will be appraised yearly, at an 'annual appraisal', to help doctors identify their educational needs and discuss performance concerns; very much a *formative process*. It is clear that in order to achieve a true picture of a doctor's performance and cover the standards set out in *Good Medical Practice*, an assessment of the practice will need to take place too, and some of the issues which will be focused on have been highlighted in the earlier chapters of this book.
- Third, every five years the information gathered at the annual appraisal stage will be passed to the GMC for the *summative 'Revalidation'* process. The GMC is quite clear that by this stage revalidation will be a 'pass or fail' situation. If the annual appraisal process has worked well, there should be no surprises.

As such, most clinical governance teams within PCOs have put a lot of emphasis on ensuring the availability of lectures and courses for the whole practice team, not just GPs and nurses. They have tried to emphasise the importance of professional development for all staff. Certainly, CHI clinical governance reviews focus on PCOs' and practices' attitudes towards the training and development of administrative staff as well as clinical staff.

Education for doctors

Getting the right balance between pursuing the medical topics that one enjoys and wishes to enhance to the full, and spending time on the weaker areas of one's knowledge can be difficult. Discovering the gaps in knowledge is also not easy. The acronyms 'DENs', or 'doctors' educational needs', and 'PUNs', or 'patients' unmet needs', are sometimes used when discussing methods of identifying one's own educational needs. Some local PCOs' clinical governance teams have changed this to be more inclusive of the whole team by coining the phrase 'personal educational needs' or 'PENs'.

This chapter sets out to identify whether practices have an atmosphere of learning.

Personal professional development

A further important dimension to this equation is one's personal interests not necessarily directly related to medical practice. Pursuing one's interests is, of course, vital for maintaining one's own sanity! Therefore, it is indirectly good for patient care also.

Such topics may have no apparent direct link to primary care, but invariably some principles are transferable. Aviation medicine and the physiology of altitude may not appear at first to be relevant to GPs other than those working for the Royal Air Force, but many patients fly abroad every year, and many are likely to be at risk from flying. A fuller understanding of which patients are at risk may make one a local expert, to be consulted frequently. An interest in medical politics, for example, may lead to a greater understanding of local and national health priorities; while aspects of management can also be transferable to the practice environment.

To help doctors get the triad of patients' needs, continuing medical education and personal interests to join up, many PCOs have produced advice folders and leaflets which encourage GPs to develop a personal professional development plan (PPDP), with aims, objectives and targets in all areas. The same principles should be followed for all practice staff, not just the clinical staff.

Personal professional development plans should also reflect the practice development plan (PDP), which in itself should reflect national and local health priorities. In this way, personal education positively influences patient outcomes.

Records

Records of educational activity will be essential for future appraisal and revalidation. No longer is it considered enough to sit snoozing at the back of a lecture theatre while a lecture is delivered, then collect a certificate at the end. A personal record of attendance must include reasons why the lecture or course was attended. This may relate to PPDP, the PDP or some other valid reason. It must also include what was gained from the lecture or course, and how this will be followed up in the future. But most importantly, it must say how it has altered your practice or how it will improve the service for patients.

Key questions

- Does the practice positively encourage education and learning for all staff?
- Are educational activities focused directly or indirectly on improved patient care?
- Is learning disseminated throughout the practice?

Suggested record of educational activity

Name: Surgery address: Date:
Title of course, lecture or meeting; book or article read
Reason for attending course, lecture or meeting (area of personal development or area of practice development addressed)
Were these adequately addressed? If not, how can they be addressed?
What were the key messages learnt?
In what way will your work or practice change as a result of this activity?
What further learning needs were discovered as a result of attending the course, lecture or meeting; or reading the book or article?
When will this need reviewing or updating?

Continuing medical education and personal professional development

	Score 1	Score 2	Score 3	Score 4	Score 5	Score 6	Score 7	Score 8	Score 9
Does the practice set aside a **budget** for educational purposes?	No			Yes. It covers vital courses that the practice expect staff to attend, but is not really sufficient to cover everybody's needs			Yes, the budget is carefully planned in line with the perceived needs within the practice development plan. It covers all members of staff, not just clinical staff. The practice will consider all requests for training and education and allocate funding depending on the relevance of the course in relation to specific criteria. These criteria are patient- and service-focused		
Does the practice have a **lead person responsible** for ensuring the educational needs of all staff are met?	No			Yes, but this person tends to focus mainly on the clinical staff only			Yes. This person ensures that the education undertaken fits in with the practice development plans as well as personal professional development plans of all staff members		

E	Are **records** kept of all educational activity?	No. The doctors keep certificates of Postgraduate Educational Allowance accredited lectures, but no other records are kept		Yes. Most courses and lectures attended are recorded in the staff members' records			Yes. Records are kept of all education and training activities, including reading and in-practice activities and meetings. The records kept show not only times and dates, but also record in what way the staff member feels that their job will be enhanced by attending the course, and in what way patients or practice will benefit (if appropriate). Further, the date that the area should be reviewed or updated		
		Score 1	Score 2	Score 3	Score 4	Score 5	Score 6	Score 7	Score 8	Score 9

Clinical staff

E	Does the practice have a programme or policy to ensure that all medical staff regularly update their knowledge and skills in **vital clinical areas**, like cardiopulmonary resuscitation and infection control?	No			Yes, but it is left very much to the individual to keep these areas updated			Yes. The practice educational lead ensures that these vital areas are constantly under review		
		Score 1	Score 2	Score 3	Score 4	Score 5	Score 6	Score 7	Score 8	Score 9
	Does the practice ensure that clinical staff maintain their skills and knowledge of more **specialised areas of service** provision – for example, running specific clinics, taking cervical smears, suturing or minor surgery skills?	No			Yes, but individuals are expected to take a lead themselves			Yes. The educational lead ensures that no service is undertaken without first ensuring that the professional has completed the appropriate accreditation course and then ensures that the necessary skills are monitored, evaluated and updated regularly		
		Score 1	Score 2	Score 3	Score 4	Score 5	Score 6	Score 7	Score 8	Score 9

		Score 1	Score 2	Score 3	Score 4	Score 5	Score 6	Score 7	Score 8	Score 9
	When staff attend courses or lectures, are they encouraged to **disseminate the learning** to others in the practice, when appropriate?	No			Yes, sometimes, but this is an area where the practice could improve			Yes. This is seen as an important part of attending courses and invariably takes place during PHCT education meetings. It usually leads to individuals becoming enthusiasts and champions for specific areas of service provision, thus benefiting the whole practice		
G	Does the practice ensure that courses attended are in line with the **practice development plan?**	No			Yes, but rarely focuses on local and national agendas			Yes. The practice development plan and most courses also focus on national and local health agendas		
G	Do the clinical staff – including the doctors – have an **annual appraisal?**	No			No, but the nurses have regular clinical supervision			Yes, all clinical staff have an annual appraisal. The practice has set up a link with a neighbouring practice to undertake co-mentoring and annual appraisal for doctors. Meanwhile, the nurses continue to undertake clinical supervision. The educational lead coordinates these activities and ensures that records are kept accordingly		

QTD MAP FBA QPA	Does the practice undertake clinical meetings where **reflection on patient care** takes place?	No				Yes, occasionally				Regular multidisciplinary meetings reflecting on patient care take place. Not only are these informative, they also help the practice formulate guidelines and protocols for service provision and help individuals to highlight areas of educational need		
		Score 1	Score 2	Score 3	Score 4	Score 5	Score 6	Score 7	Score 8	Score 9		

Reception and administrative staff

		Score 1	Score 2	Score 3	Score 4	Score 5	Score 6	Score 7	Score 8	Score 9
G	Does the practice have a policy to ensure the **professional development** of reception and administrative staff?	No			There is no written policy, but reception and administrative staff are encouraged to go on courses also			Yes, there is a written policy. The staff are valued and this is seen as an important part of the practice's employment policy. The practice sees this as a good way of helping retain staff		
G	Do the staff have **annual appraisals** in which educational and developmental needs are discussed?	No			Yes, but these are not recorded and not really appreciated by the staff			Yes, this is seen as a vital part of the whole staff and education agenda. The needs of the individual as well as the needs of the practice are discussed and formally recorded. Targets for educational and training requirements are set and monitored		

Comments and notes:

Significant event monitoring

(there are more questions relating to significant event monitoring in Chapter 9)

QTD MAP FBA QPA	Does the practice have regular meetings where **significant events** – positive and untoward – are part of the educational agenda?	No, there is no significant event monitoring system			There is a significant event monitoring system, but this does not form part of the educational agenda			Yes, there is a significant event monitoring system, which is well publicised and used. It is seen by *all* staff, especially the clinical staff, as an essential learning tool		
		Score 1	Score 2	Score 3	Score 4	Score 5	Score 6	Score 7	Score 8	Score 9

Comments and notes:

Total score, count the number of criteria scoring 1 and place the total in the first box, then the number scoring 2 and place in the second box and continue with scores 3, 4, 5, 6, 7, 8 and 9	The areas scoring 1, 2 or 3 **urgently** need to be put in place or need significant improvement			The areas scoring 4, 5 or 6 need reviewing and improving			The areas which are working well score 7, 8 or 9. Can the principles of these systems be transferred to other areas of practice work?		
Total scores	Score 1	Score 2	Score 3	Score 4	Score 5	Score 6	Score 7	Score 8	Score 9

L = legal requirement
G = considered good practice
MAP = Membership of the RCGP by Assessment of Performance

ToS = contractual or in Terms of Service
QTD = Quality Team Development
QTD = Quality Team Development

E = essential for revalidation
QPA = Quality Practice Award
FBA = Fellowship of the RCGP by Assessment of Performance

14

Patient and service user involvement

Background

No book on the quality of general practice written in the 21st century can be without a chapter on how patients are involved in practice development. Throughout the various chapters there has been reference to the fact that practices offering the highest quality of care do consult patients, service users and carers and support groups about services and facilities. This concluding chapter assesses practices' willingness to consult those that use the services.

The government's NHS Plan certainly sets out the challenge to all NHS providers to include patients in discussion around treatment of services. CHI has patient and service user involvement as one of its seven pillars of clinical governance, and certainly an assessment of how NHS organisations obtain patients' views forms part of the CHI clinical governance review. Likewise, CHI seeks the opinion of patients and service users about the services provided by the organisation they are about to review, and that includes general practices.

It is fair to say that most practices have found this area challenging. It is not easy to get patients to volunteer, and some practices find that those who do volunteer have 'an axe to grind' or ulterior motive for doing so. Some practices, however, have set up successful patient participation or liaison groups, and found their input invaluable.

Another successful way to get useful input from patients is to consult small groups about a specific area of service provision, for example approaching diabetic patients about the running of the diabetic service at the practice. The practice should have a clear focus on what it wishes to achieve by this discussion process and make it clear that it is a short-term project with an end point.

Self-help groups, local branches of national associations and patient advocacy groups are also willing to offer advice about the working of the practice; disability groups are a good example.

Carers should also be considered for input into services. If a practice is able to set up a carers support group, then not only will it receive invaluable advice about the care of some of the most dependent patients, but also it will be able to use this as a platform to advise the carers about the appropriate use of the practice and the most appropriate professional to contact when help is needed. Encouraging other service providers to engage with the group will make the feedback to the practice even more valuable.

Patient surveys

There are several questionnaires now available specifically to ask patients their views about the practice. Two examples are GPAS (General Practice Assessment Survey) and IPQ (Improving Practice Questionnaire).

GPAS was developed in 1998 by the National Primary Care Research and Development Centre, University of Manchester (www.npcrdc.man.ac.uk) and has been well validated. The details of this validation were published by Ramsay et al.[1] in 2000 and Campbell et al. in 2001.[2] It asks patients and service users questions about many of the areas covered in this book, including access, continuity of care, communication, receptionists, interpersonal care and doctor's knowledge about the patient, as well as referral outside the practice, nursing and overall satisfaction. The questionnaire and full details about using it can be found on the website www.gpas.co.uk.

IPQ is being used by over 30 PCTs, and, once again, is well validated. Over 80 000 patients have completed the questionnaire. It also focuses on access and availability of professionals, health promotion activities, behaviour of the receptionists and interpersonal skills of the doctor.[3] CHI uses IPQ to seek the views of patients and service users before carrying out a clinical governance review, and a modified version of IPQ to assess services of dentists, opticians and other professions allied to medicine.

Key questions

- Is the practice committed to involving patients, service users and carers in the development of service provision?
- Do patients, service users and carers feel that they are involved in practice improvements?

References

1 Ramsay J et al. (2000) Family Practice. **17**: 372–9.
2 Campbell J et al. (2001) Quality in Health Care. **10**: 90–5.
3 Greco M (2001) Use patient feedback to implement the NHS Plan. Primary Care Report. **3**(12): 24–6.

Patient and service user involvement

	Score 1	Score 2	Score 3	Score 4	Score 5	Score 6	Score 7	Score 8	Score 9
Does the practice have a **patient participation or liaison group** of any kind?	No, this has not been considered			No, but this has been considered and there are plans to develop such a group			Yes. The group has been running for some time and has been instrumental in suggesting practice improvements. It has also been involved in the implementation of many policies affecting patients and service users		
Does the practice discuss development of **specific disease-focused services** with those suffering from the disease?	No			Yes, but the views were not taken into consideration			Yes. The local branches of some national organisations have been consulted about a number of specific services as well as those on the practice list. Significant benefit was felt to have been gained from doing so		
Has the practice **sought patients' and users' views** about the practice and the services?	No.			Once, a while ago, and few changes were made as a result of the views expressed			Yes. The practice makes every effort to seek patients' and service users' views about the whole way the practice delivers services. Appropriate changes and additions to services are always considered		

		Score 1	Score 2	Score 3	Score 4	Score 5	Score 6	Score 7	Score 8	Score 9
	Has the practice ever asked patients and service users their views about the **practice buildings and facilities?**	No			Yes, a few changes were made as a result			Yes. Several groups as well as patients and service users were involved in the design of the building, and before any building developments go ahead, patients and users are consulted		
MAP FBA QPA	Has the practice ever used **patient questionnaires** to obtain views from patients and service users?	No			Yes, a while ago			Yes. The practice regularly uses questionnaires to obtain patients' views about the practice		
	Has the practice asked patients, service users and carers about the quality of the **practice leaflet?**	No			Yes, a long time ago. Few changes were made as a result of the feedback			Yes. Patients and service users made a valuable contribution and many changes were made as a result of the feedback, for example the leaflet is now available in large font sizes and Braille		

Does the practice encourage **patients to express their views** spontaneously?	No			Yes. There is a suggestions box available for patients to put comments in. It is rarely, if ever, used			Yes. The practice has a specific leaflet expressing how patients can give feedback. Further, all comments made are followed up and the patient contacted to ask for further comment if appropriate. This is particularly the case for informal grumbles and complaints		
	Score 1	Score 2	Score 3	Score 4	Score 5	Score 6	Score 7	Score 8	Score 9

Does the practice involve patients and service users in **monitoring specific services?**	No			Yes, but only occasionally. Monitoring is usually done without patients being aware that it happens			Yes. Patients with specific problems are asked about the service as part of the monitoring process. Such patients are always informed of the outcome of the audit or monitoring process, especially if it results in a significant change in the service		
	Score 1	Score 2	Score 3	Score 4	Score 5	Score 6	Score 7	Score 8	Score 9

Does the practice have a **support group** specifically for **carers?**	No			Yes, but it is not very active and the practice doesn't give very much support			Yes. This is well run, very active and is used for educational as well as support purposes		
	Score 1	Score 2	Score 3	Score 4	Score 5	Score 6	Score 7	Score 8	Score 9

Total score, count the number of criteria scoring 1 and place the total in the first box, then the number scoring 2 and place in the second box and continue with scores 3, 4, 5, 6, 7, 8 and 9	The areas scoring 1, 2 or 3 **urgently** need to be put in place or need significant improvement			The areas scoring 4, 5 or 6 need reviewing and improving			The areas which are working well score 7, 8 or 9. Can the principles of these systems be transferred to other areas of practice work?		
	Score 1	Score 2	Score 3	Score 4	Score 5	Score 6	Score 7	Score 8	Score 9
Total scores									

L = legal requirement
G = considered good practice
MAP = Membership of the RCGP by Assessment of Performance

ToS = contractual or in Terms of Service
QTD = Quality Team Development
QPA = Quality Practice Award

E = essential for revalidation
QPA = Quality Practice Award
FBA = Fellowship of the RCGP by Assessment of Performance

Index